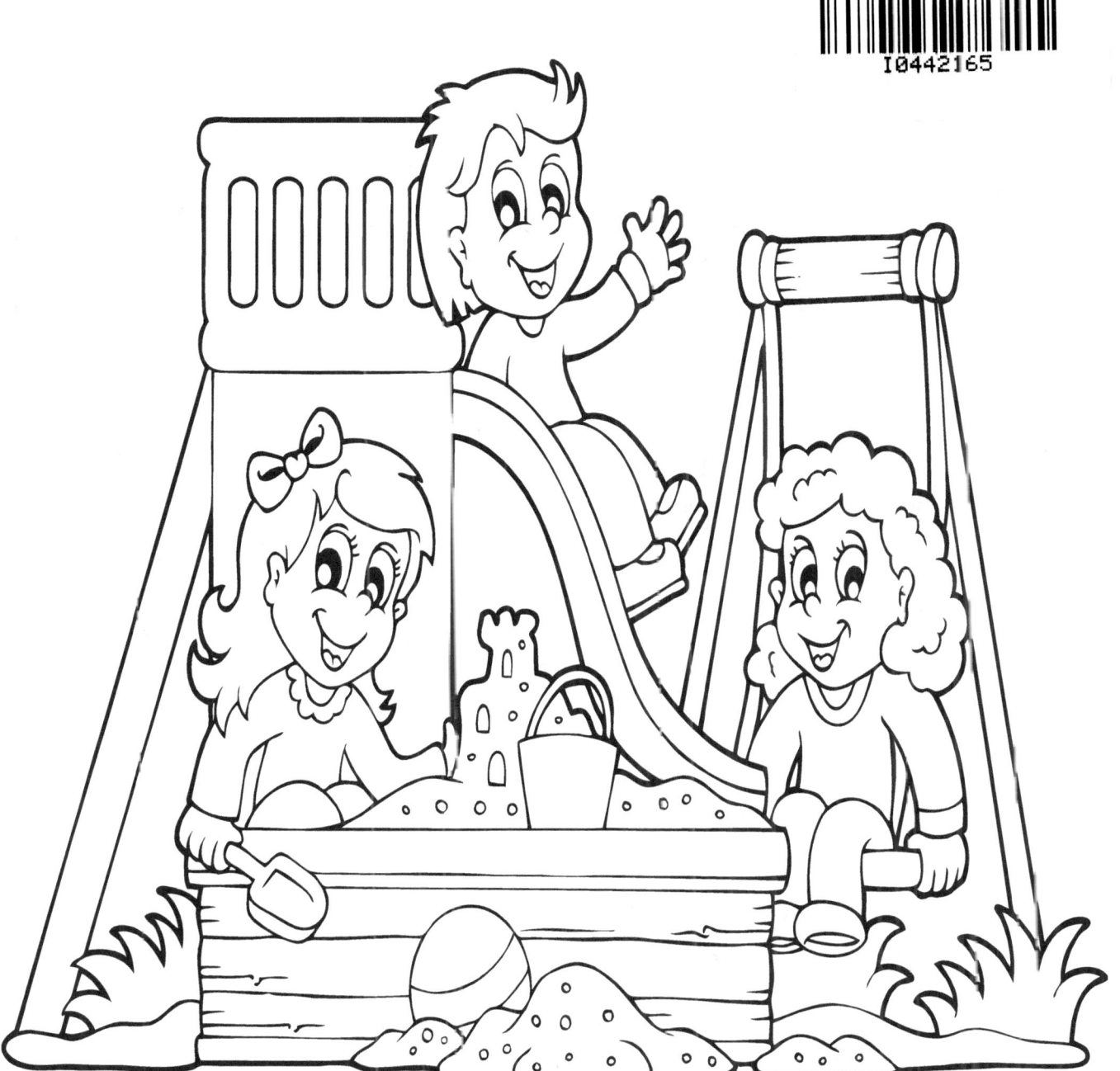

This book belongs to:

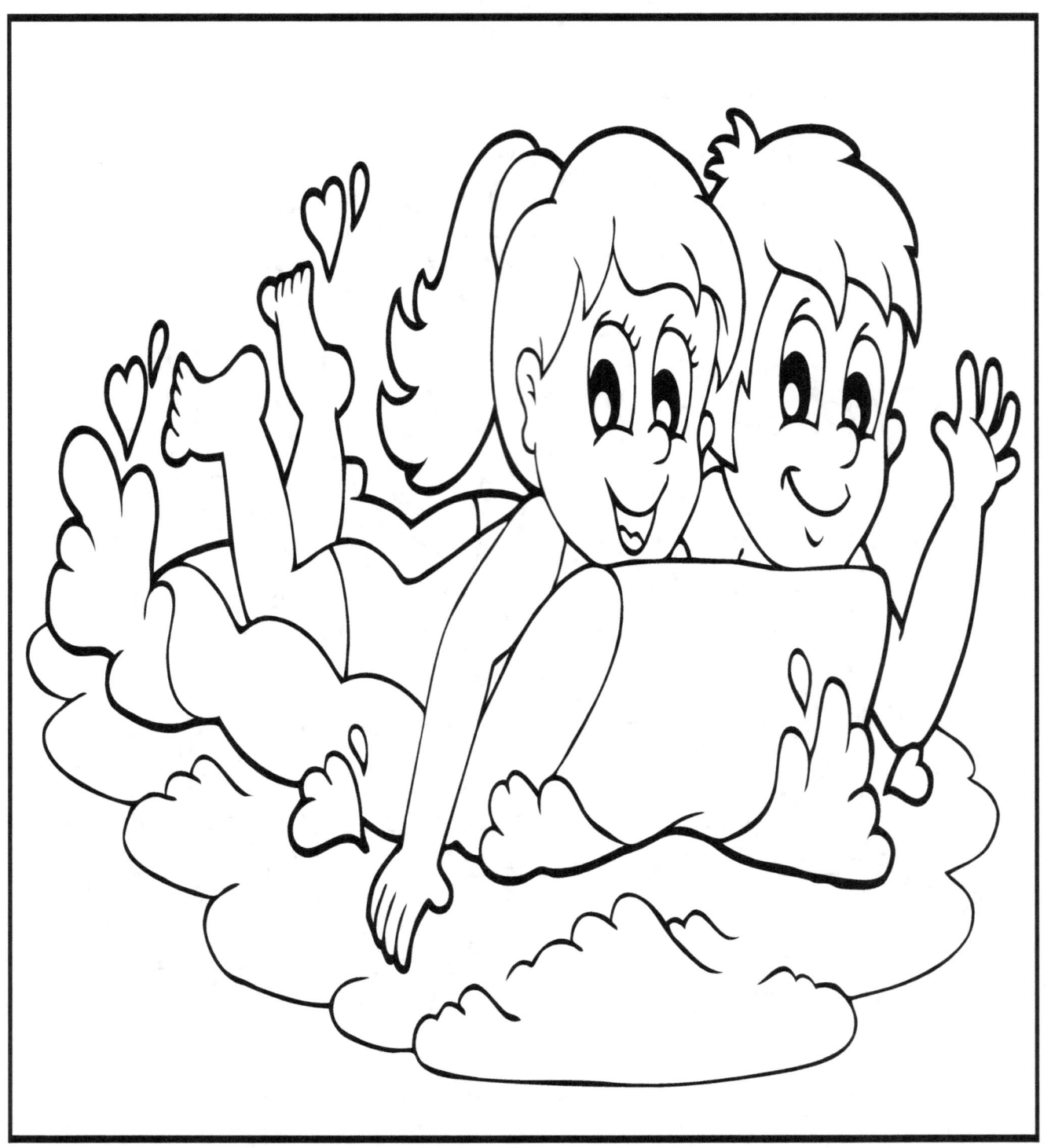

Copyright ©2016 Mary Lou Brown & Sandy Mahony

Fit Kids Have Fun

Coloring Book

Mary Lou Brown
Sandy Mahony

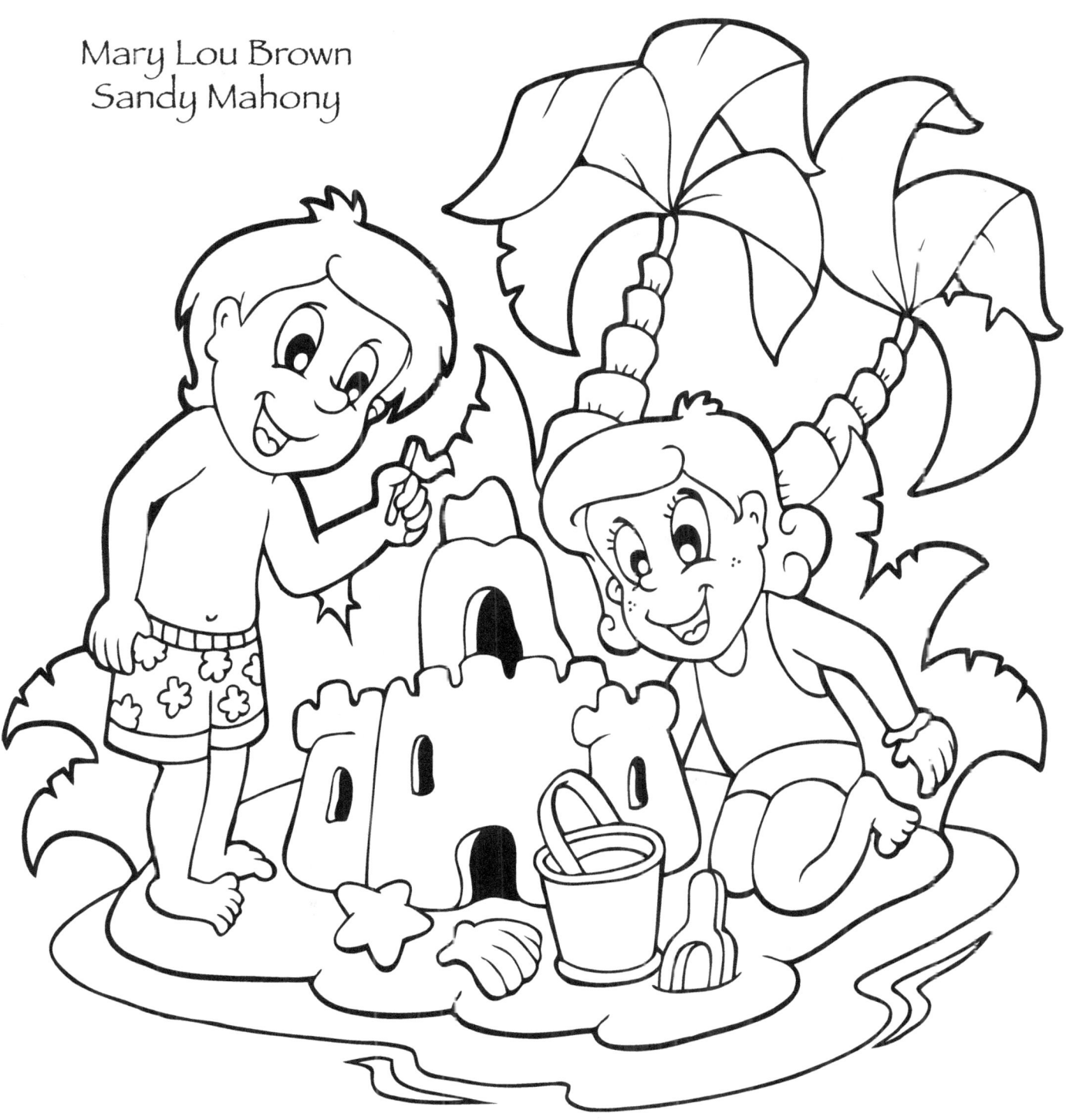

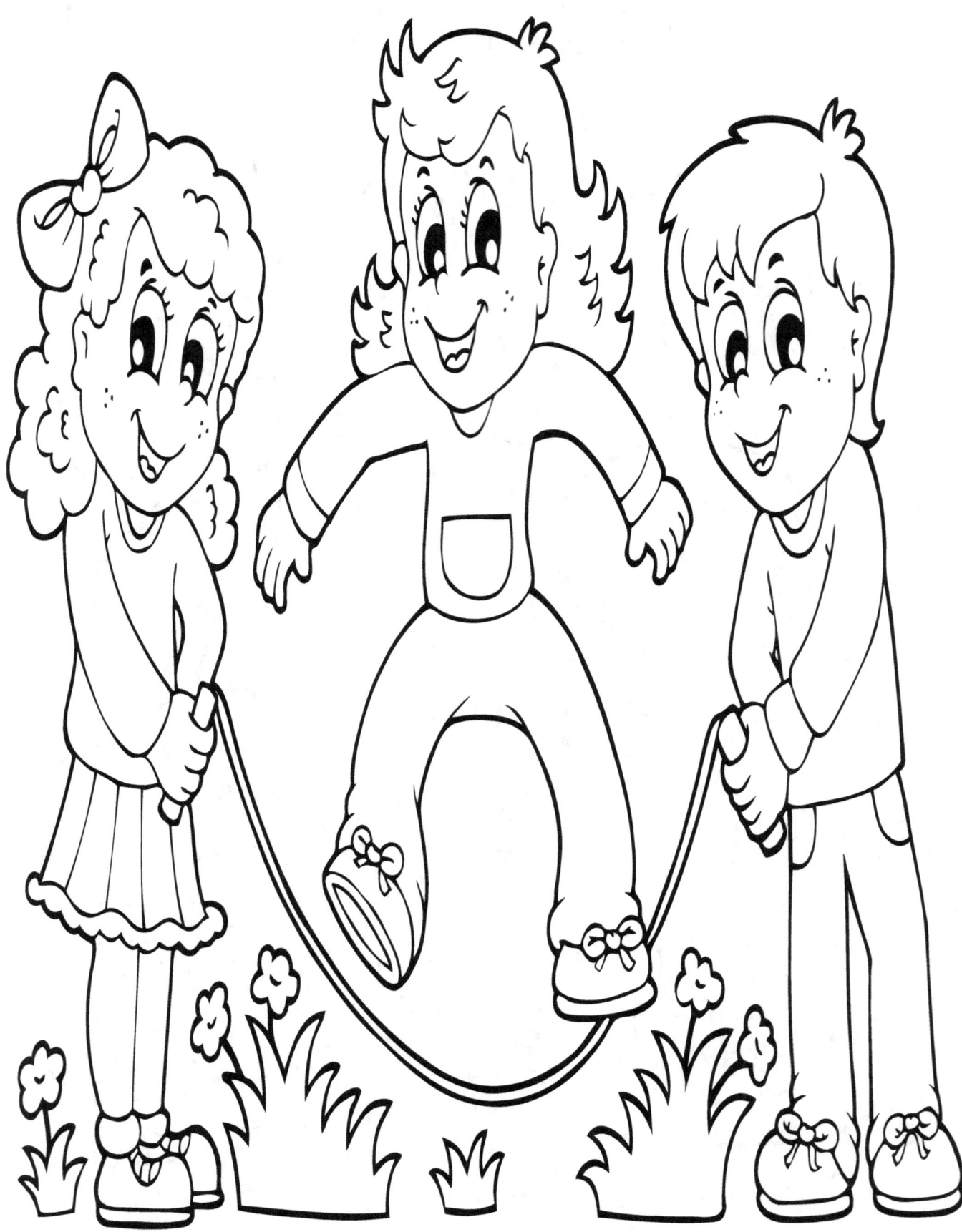

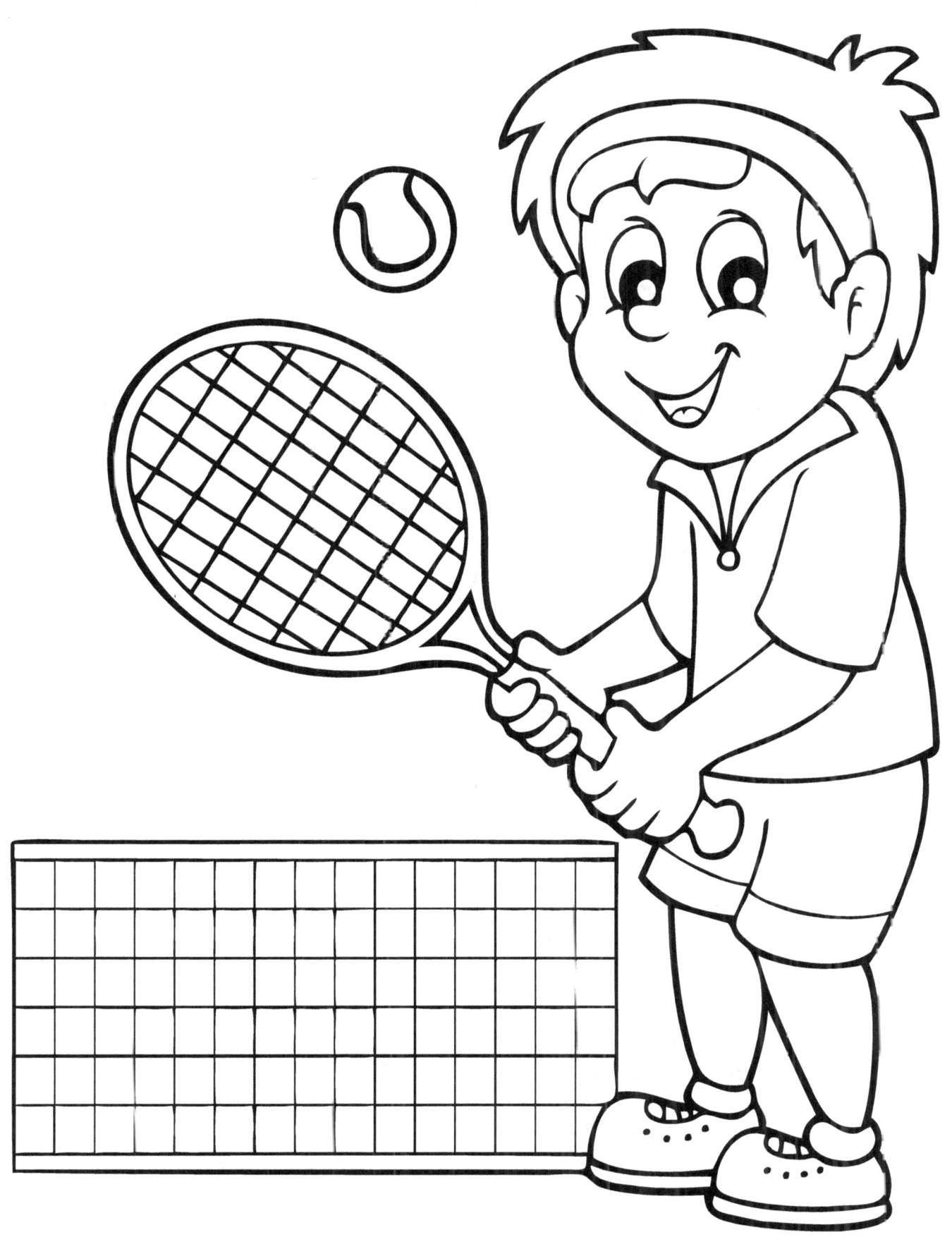

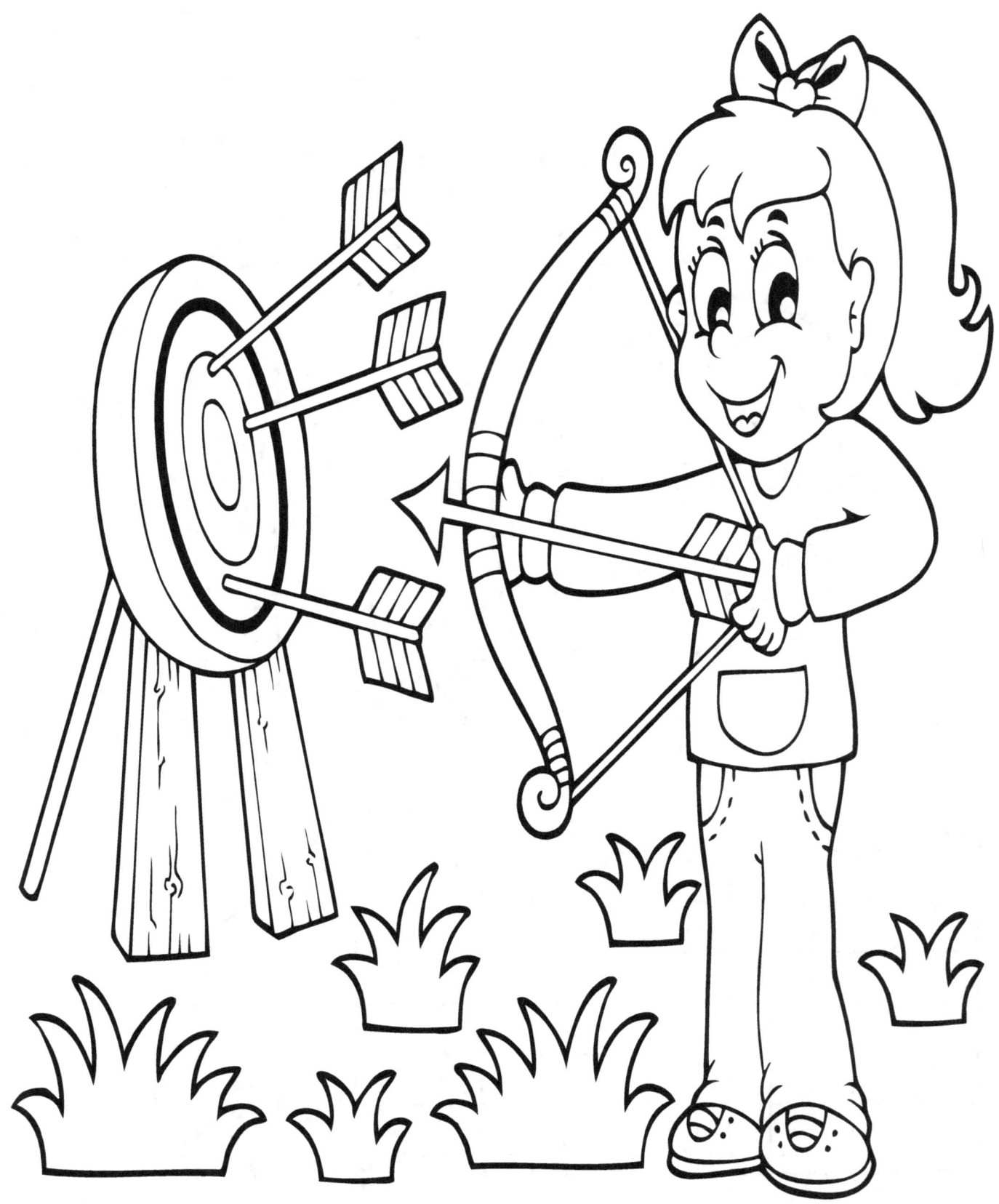

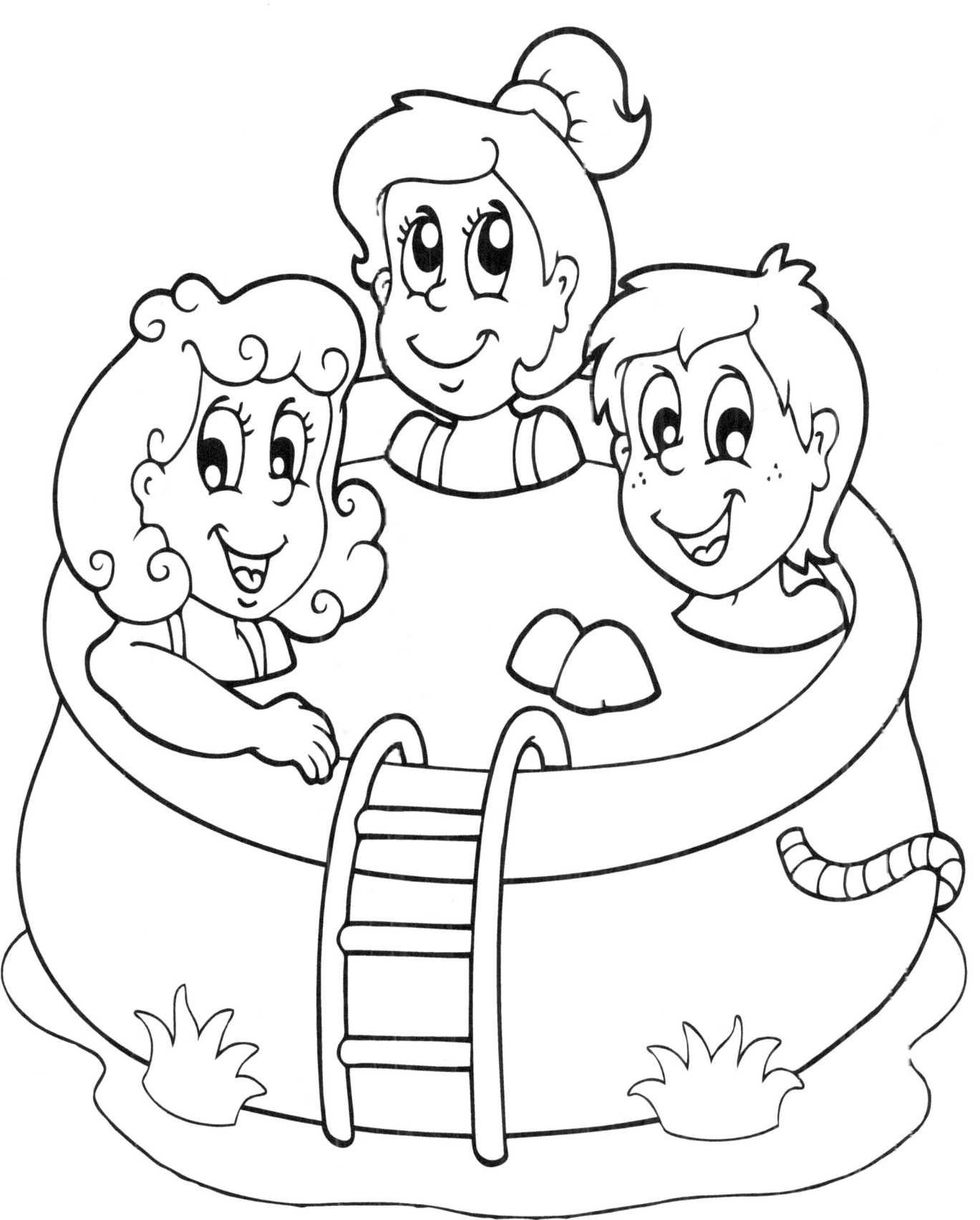

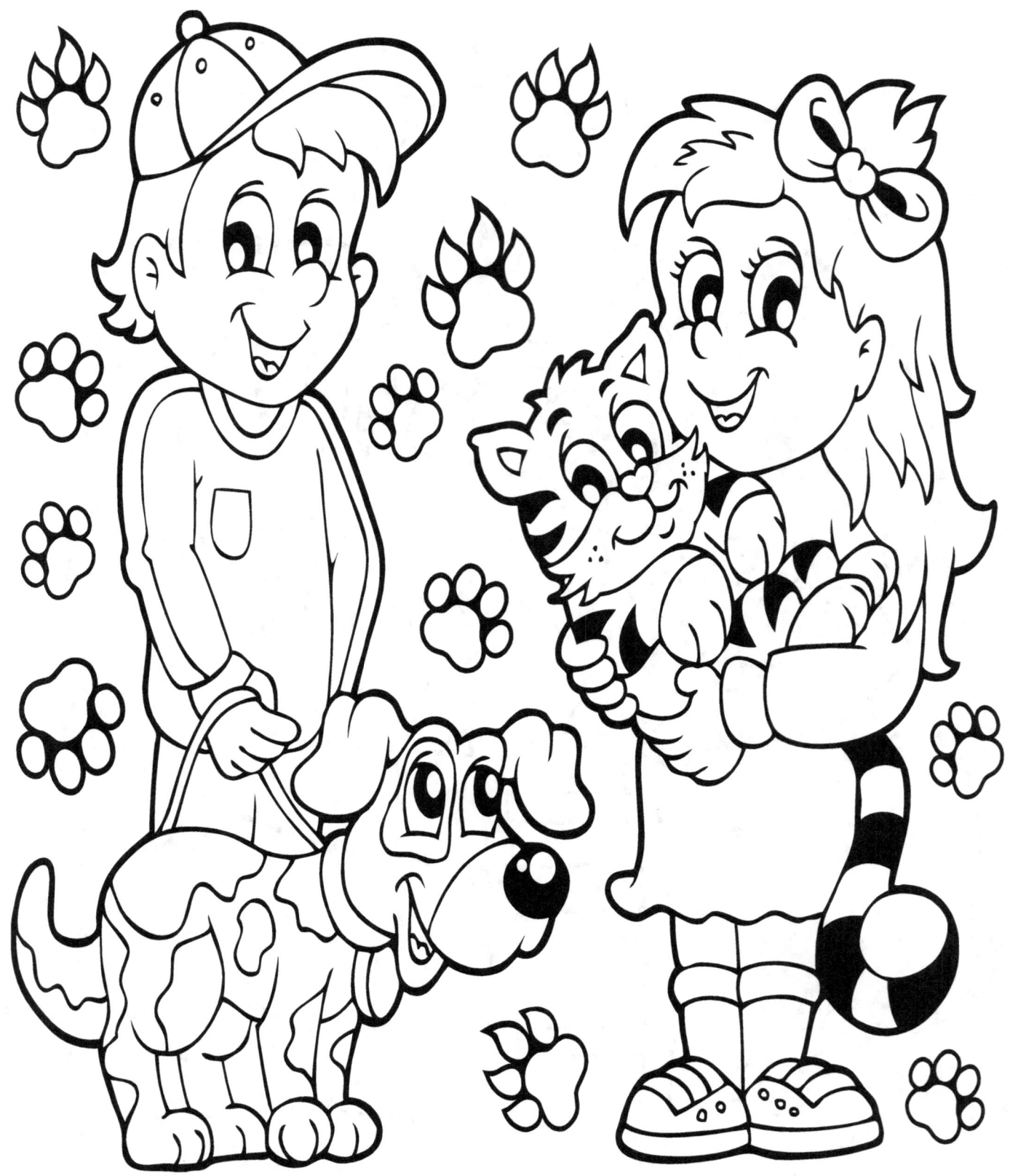

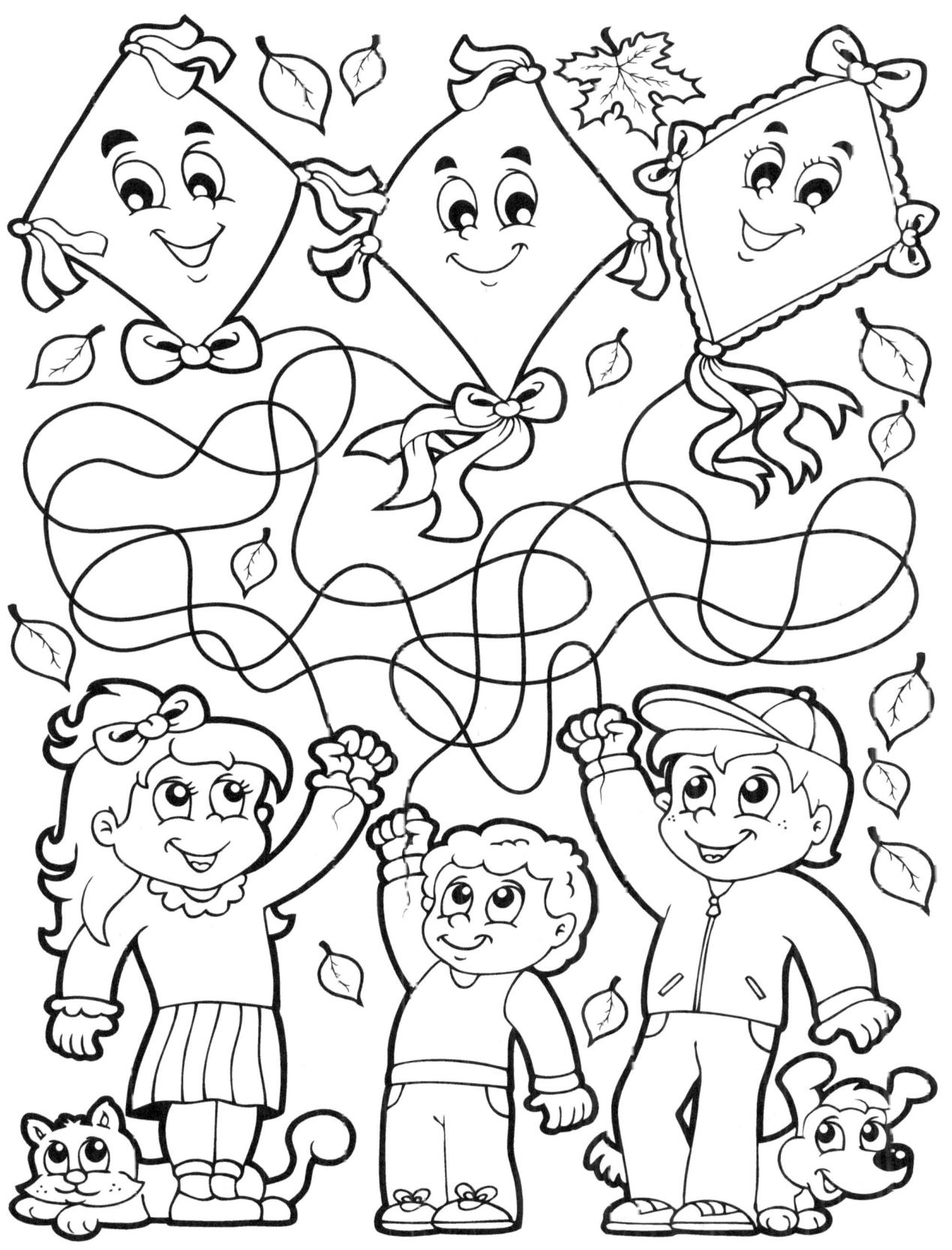

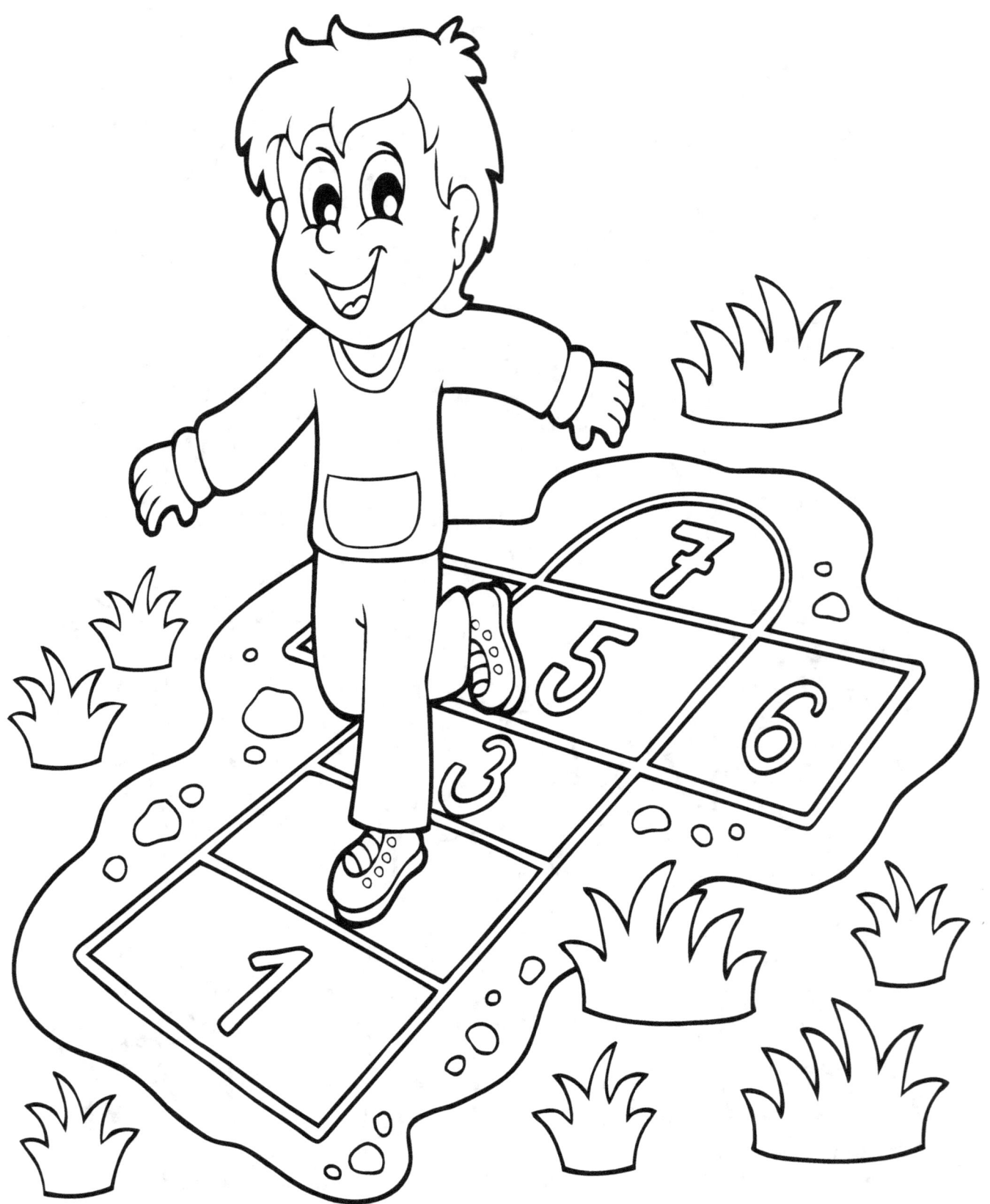

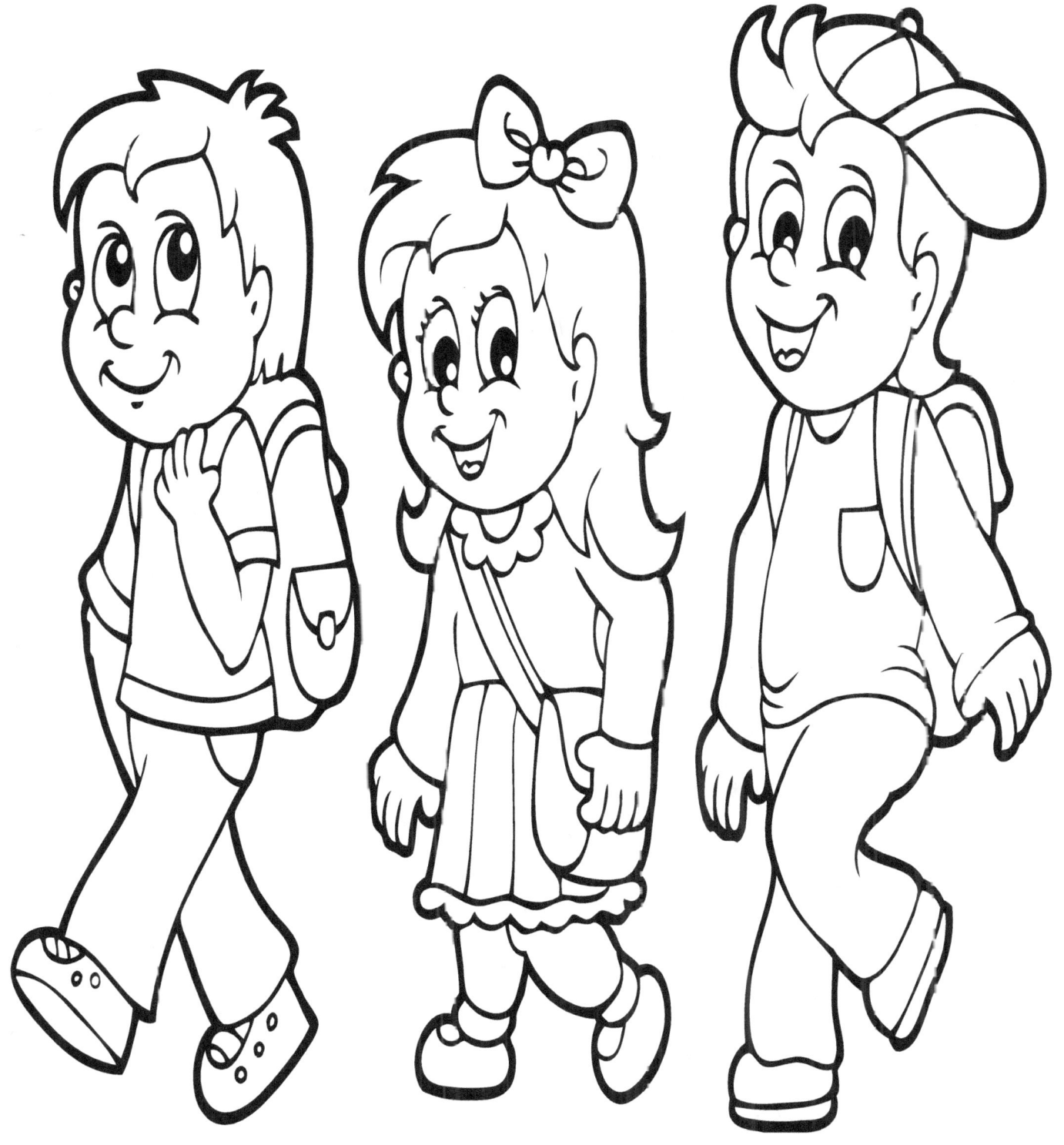

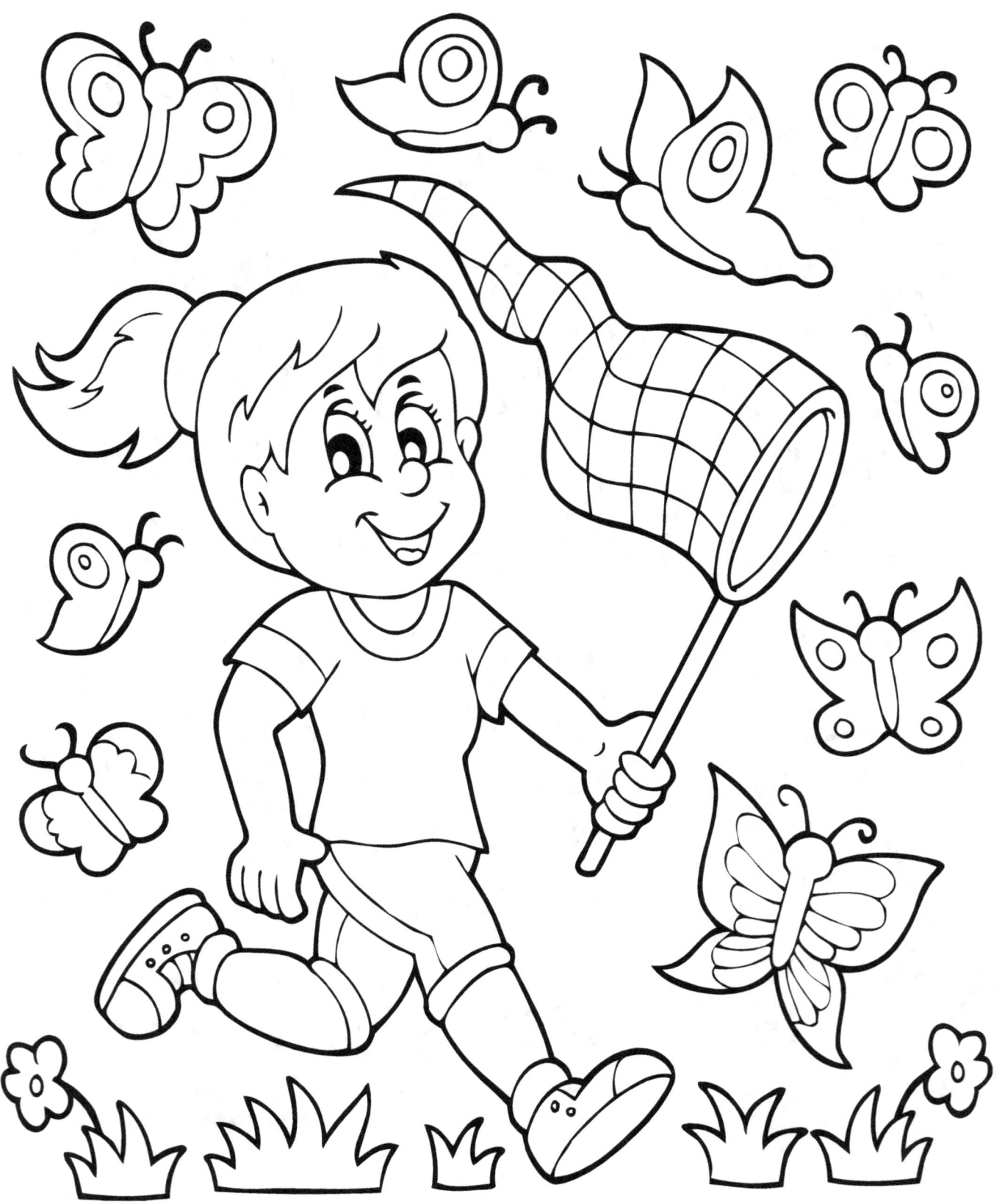

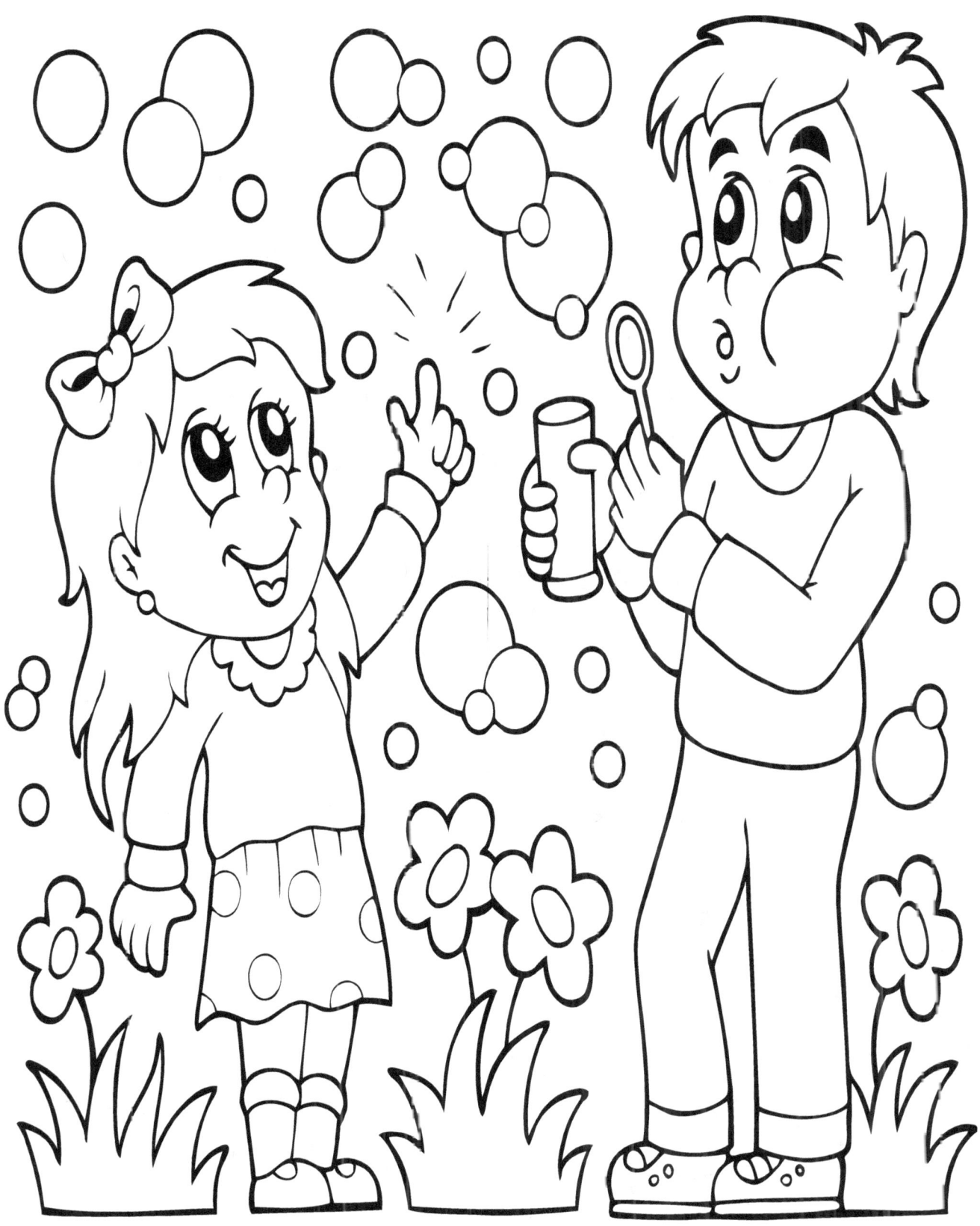

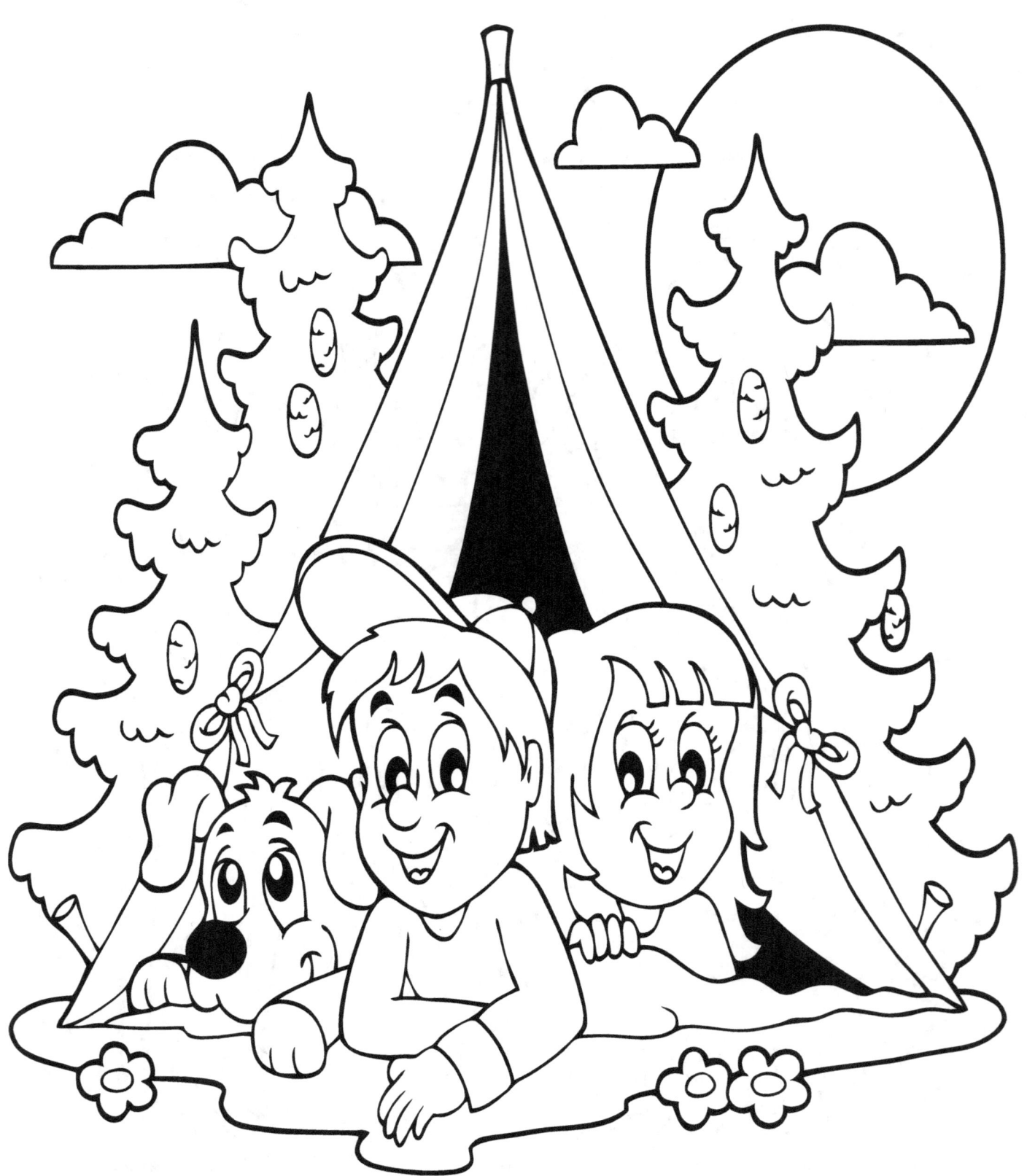

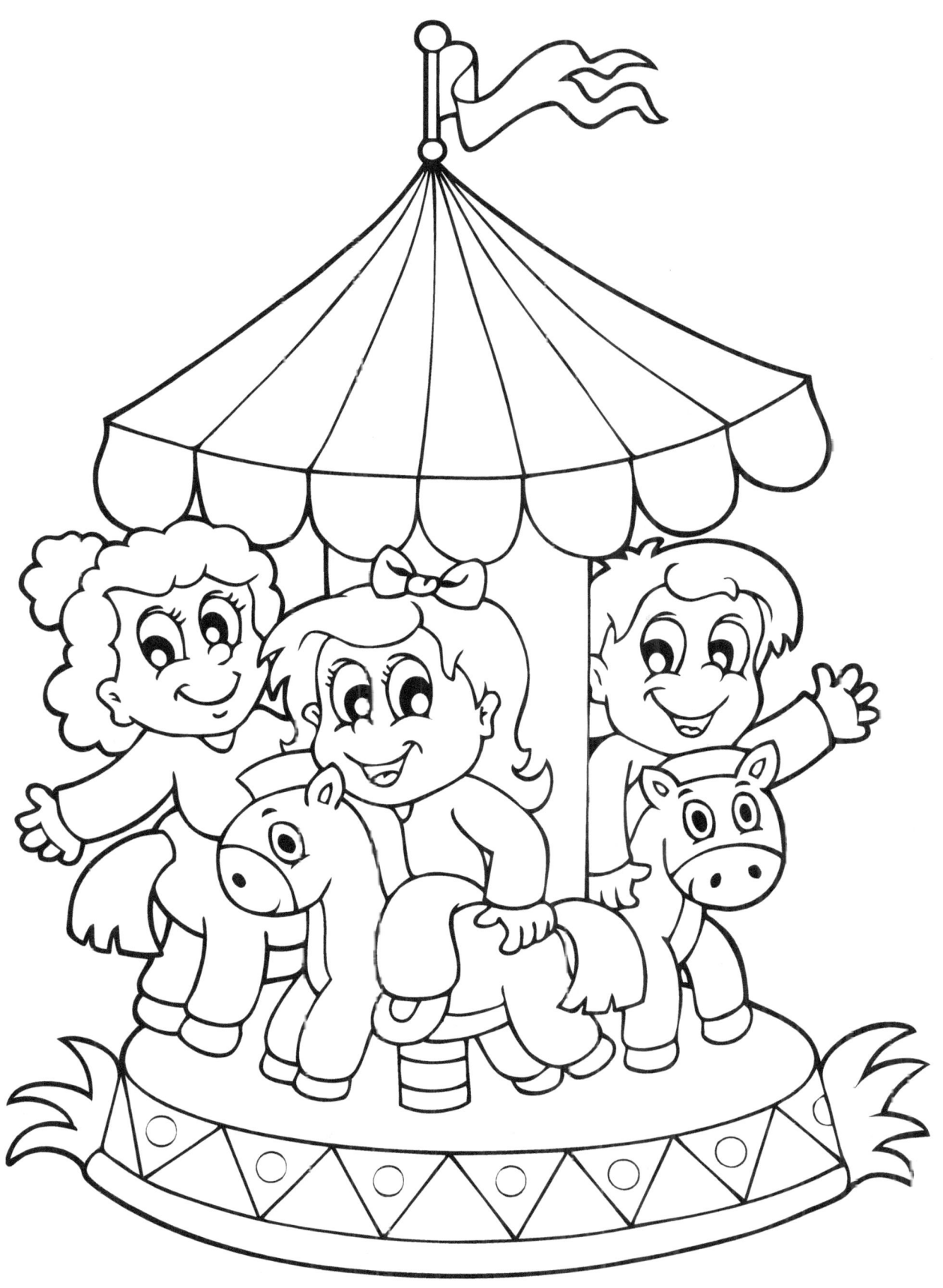

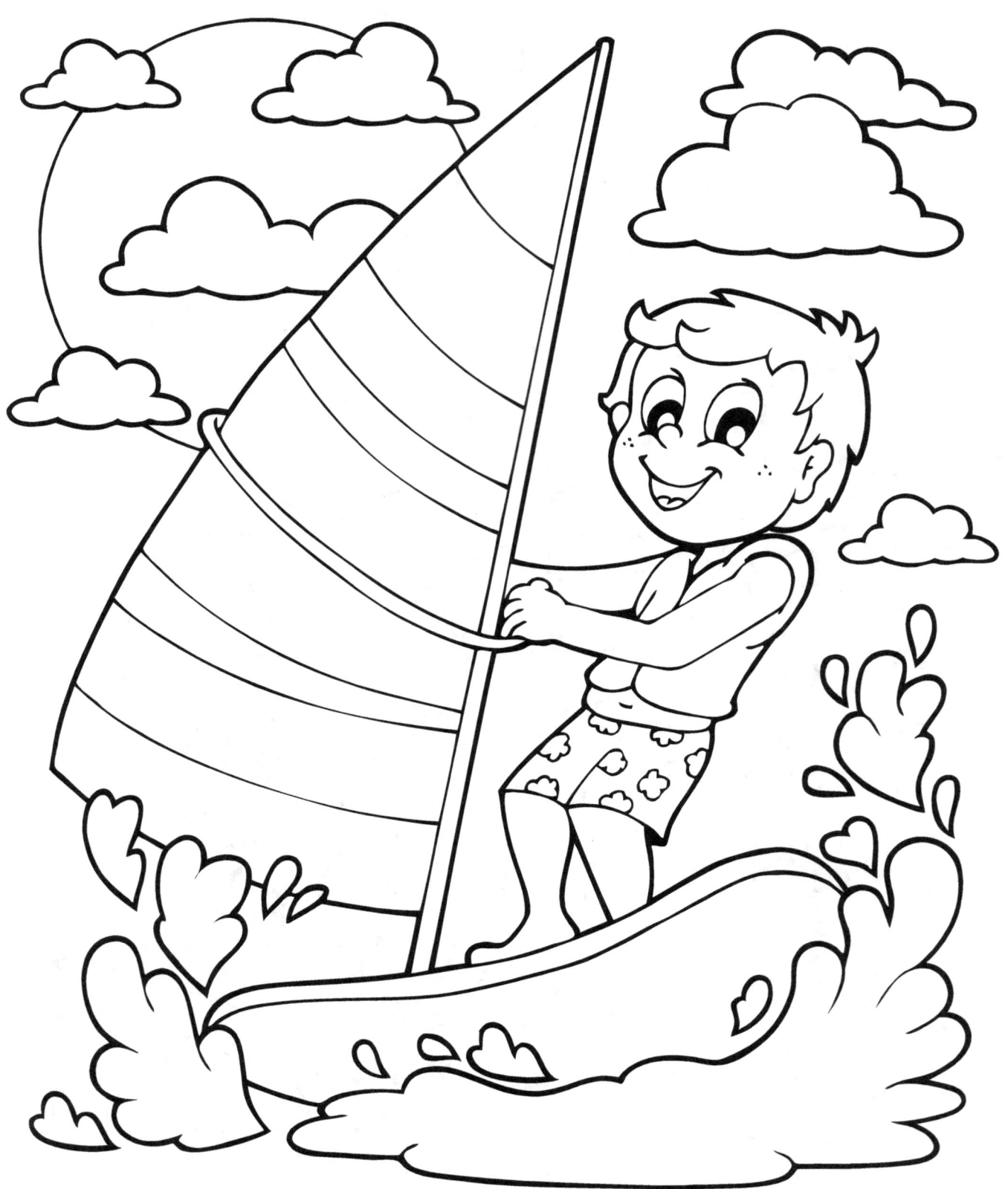

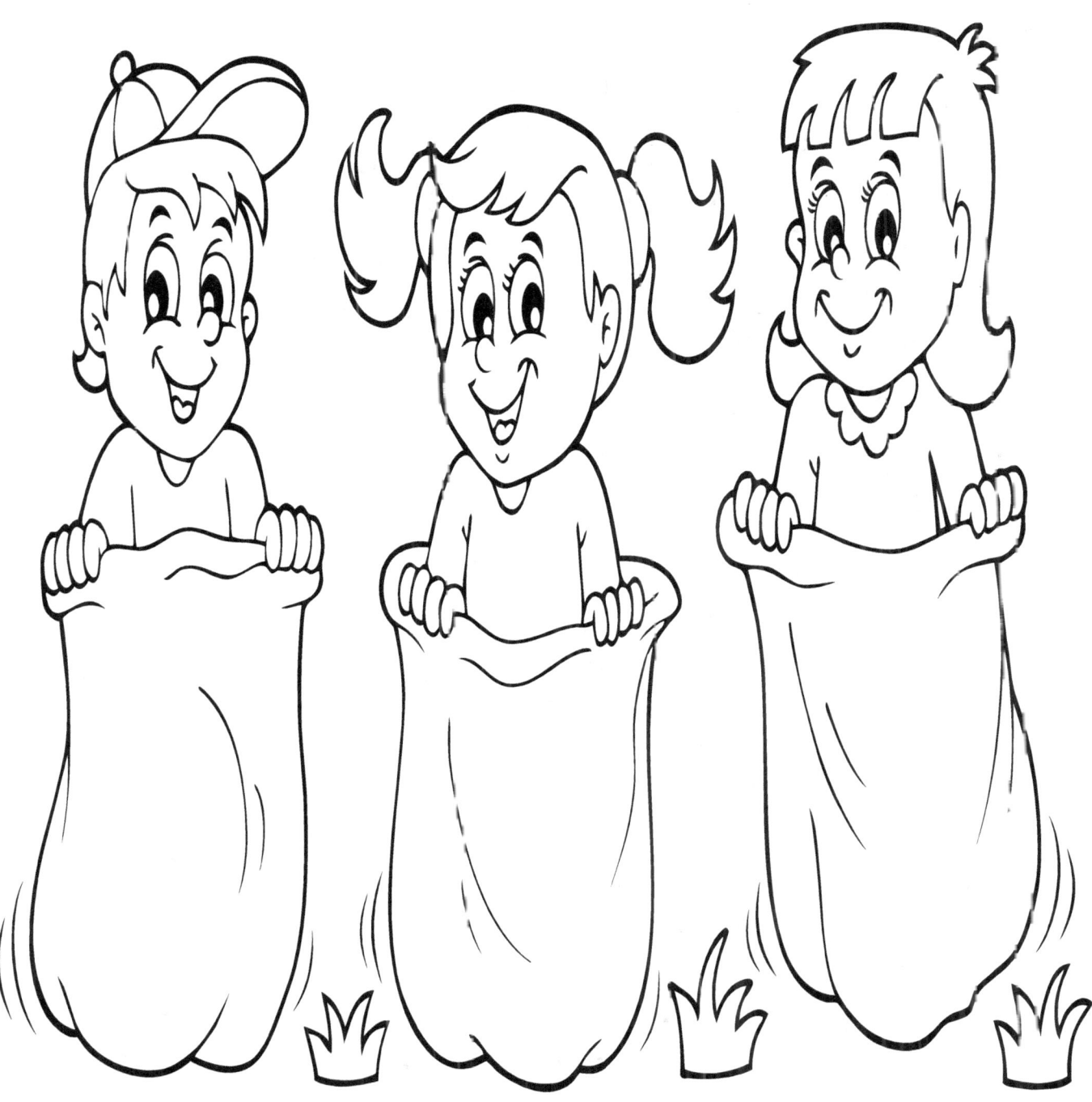

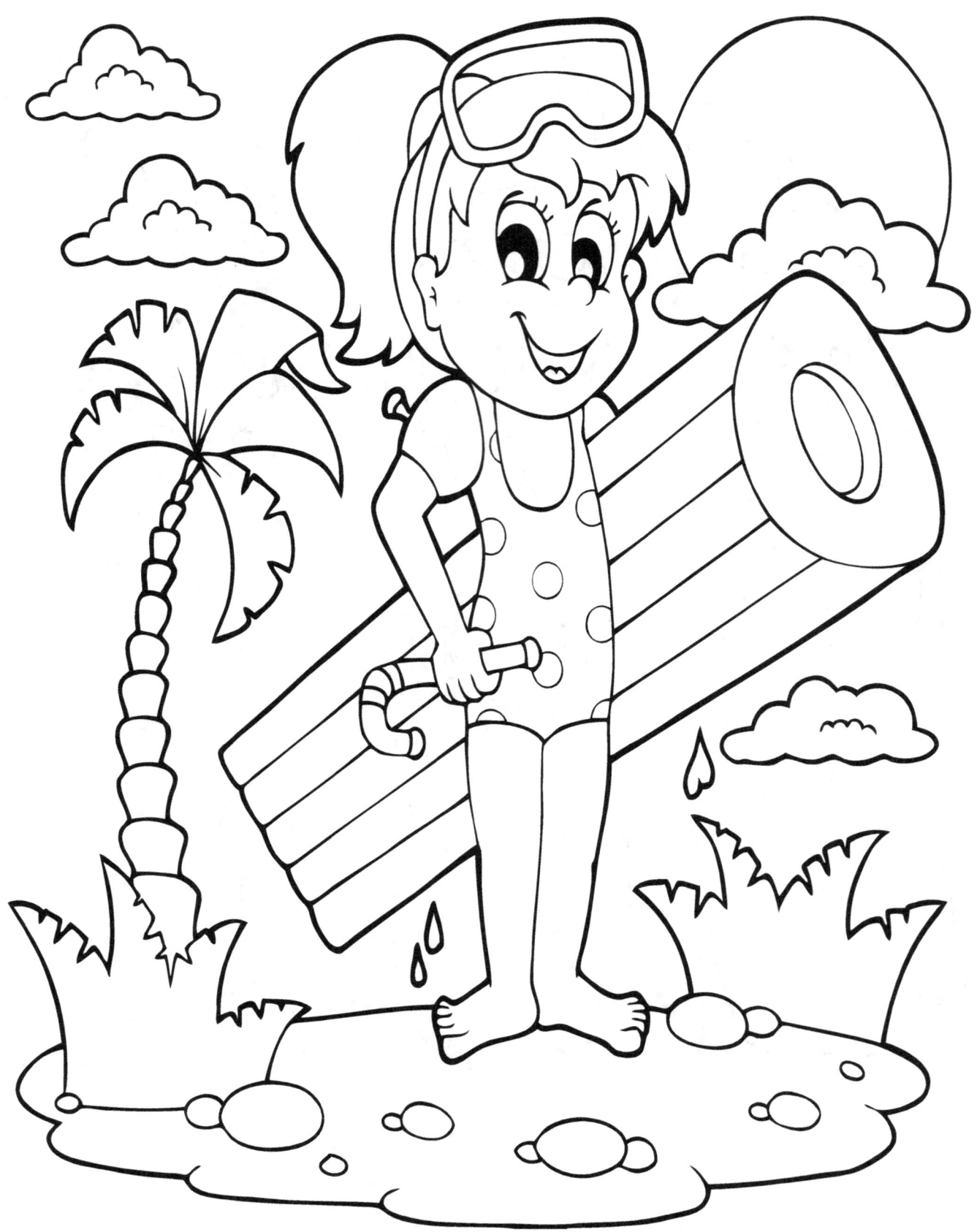

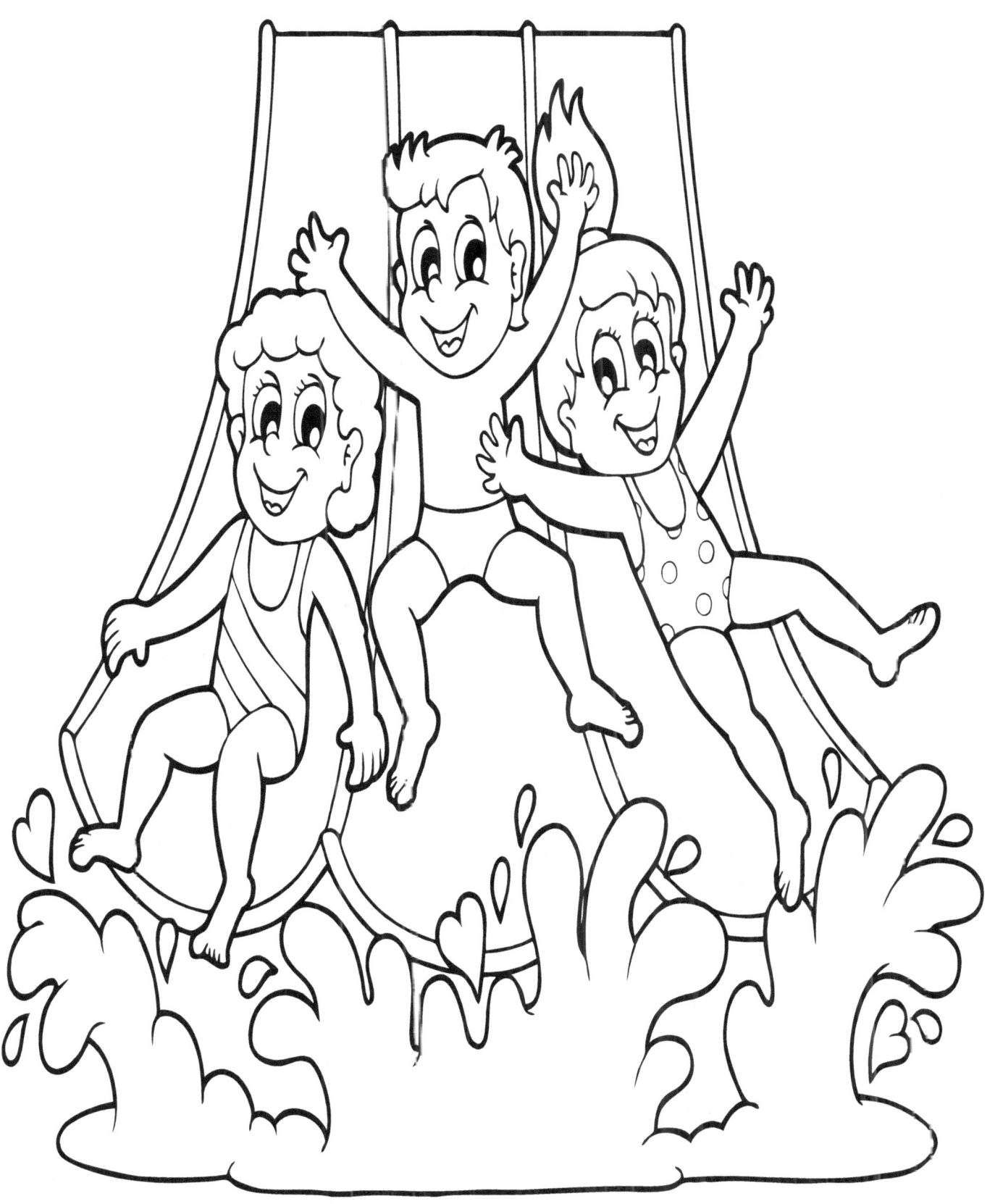

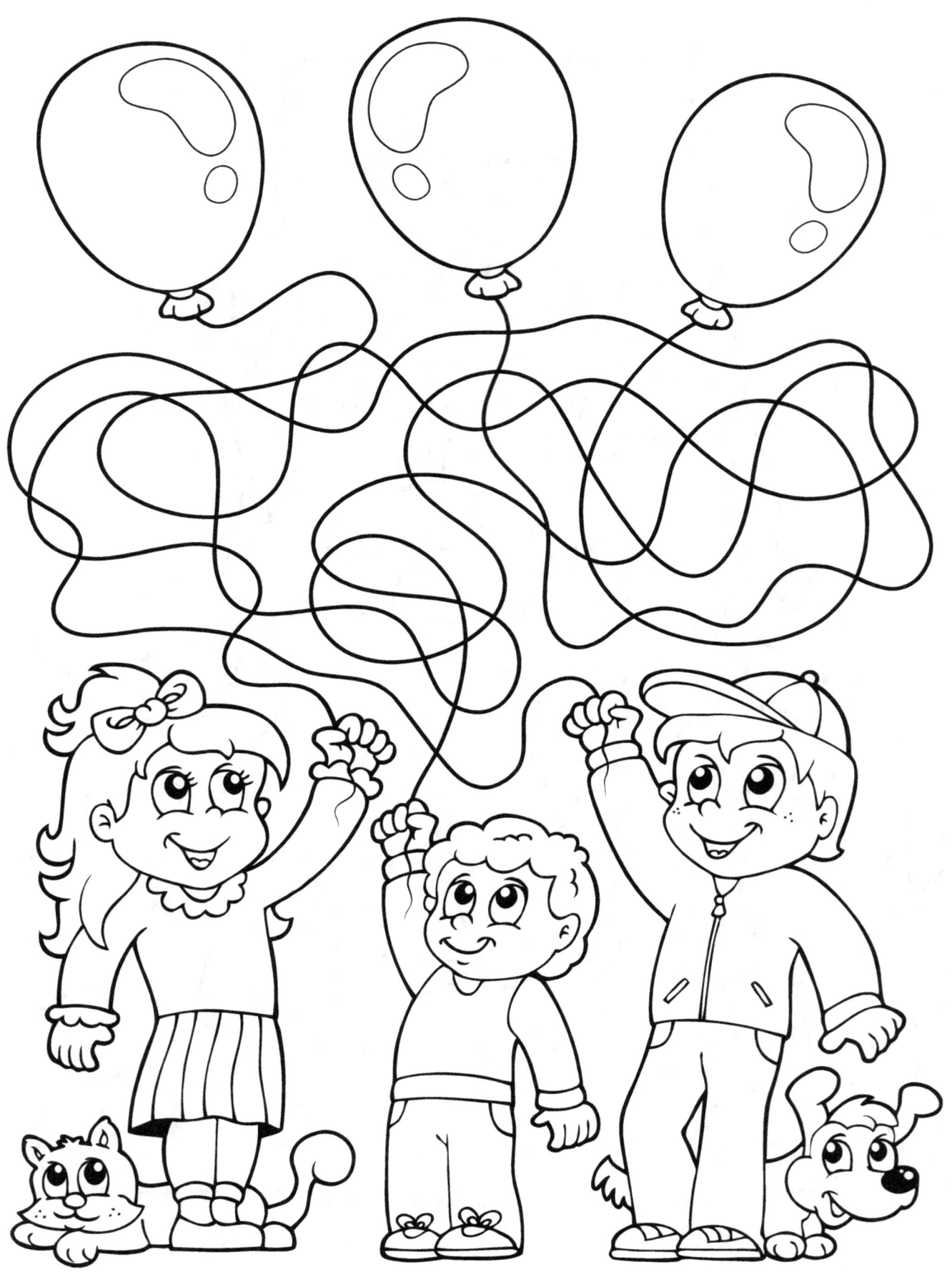

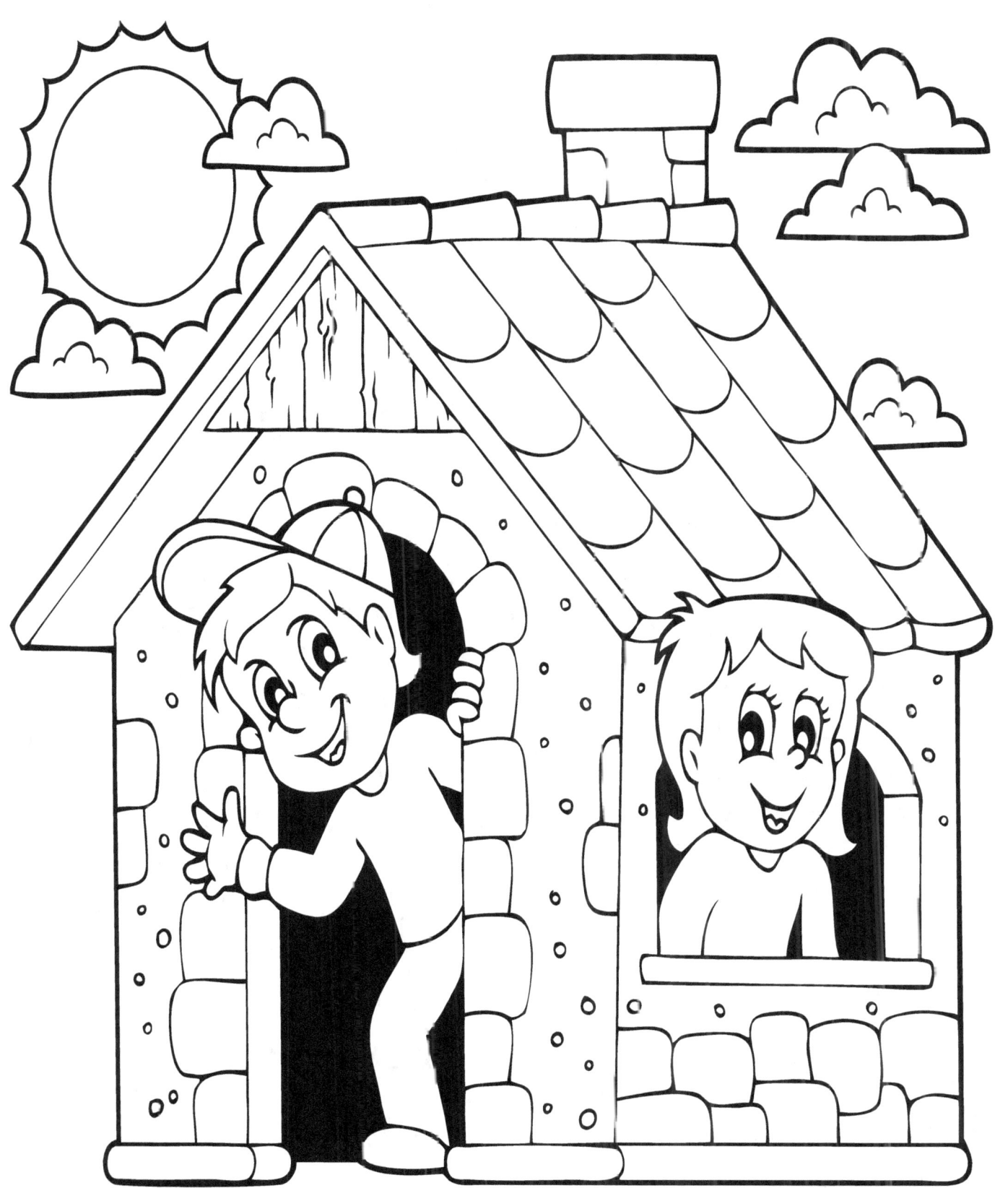

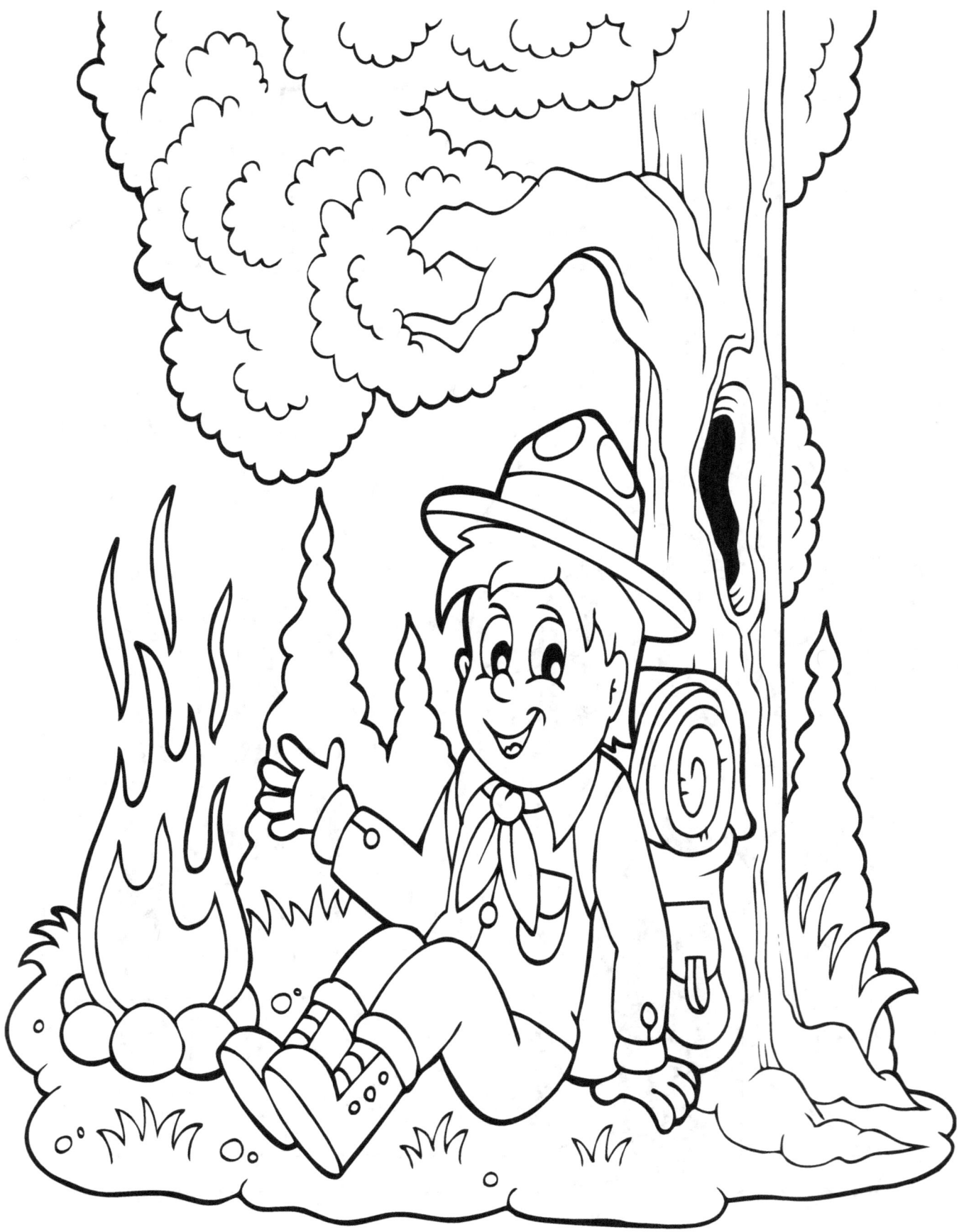

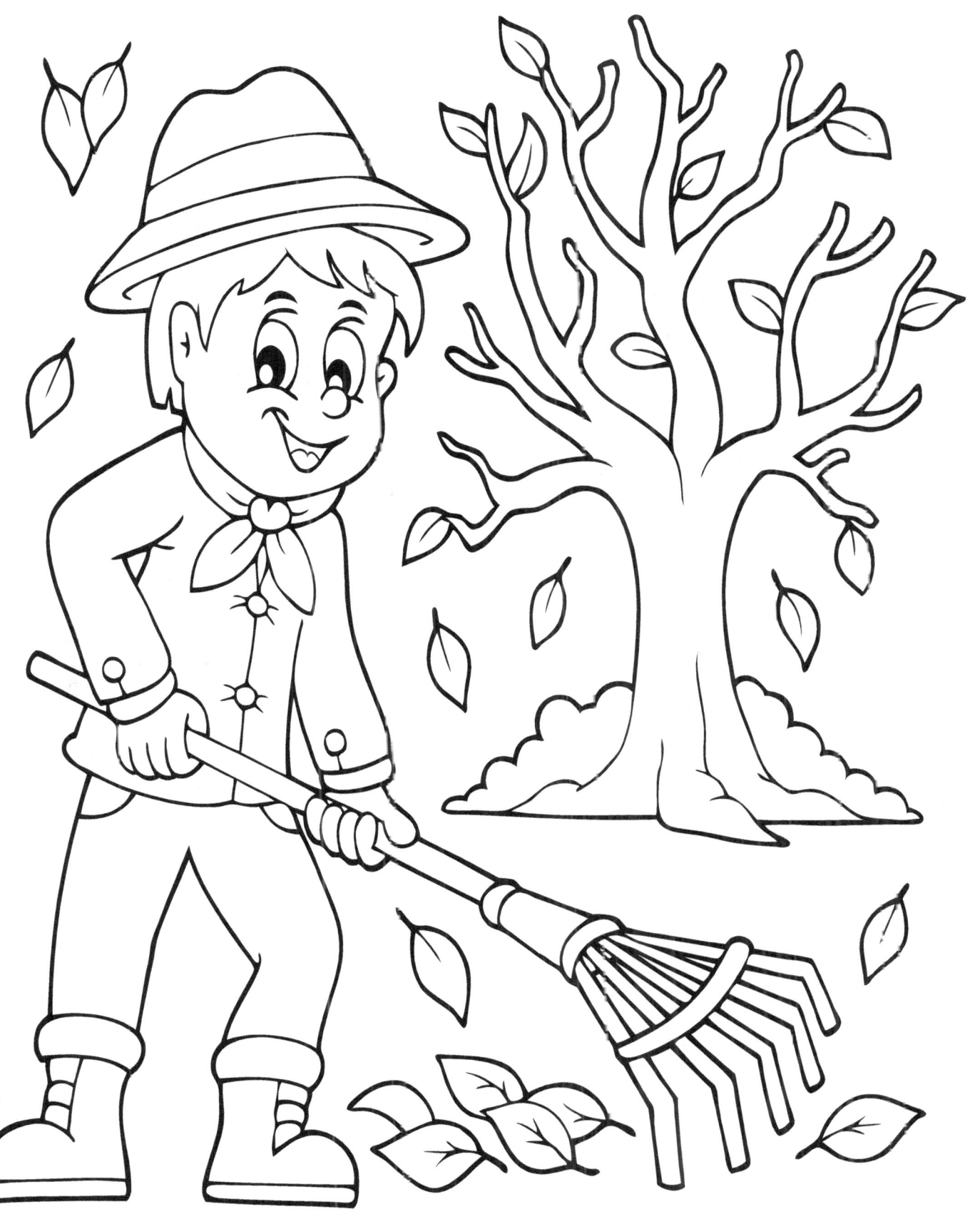

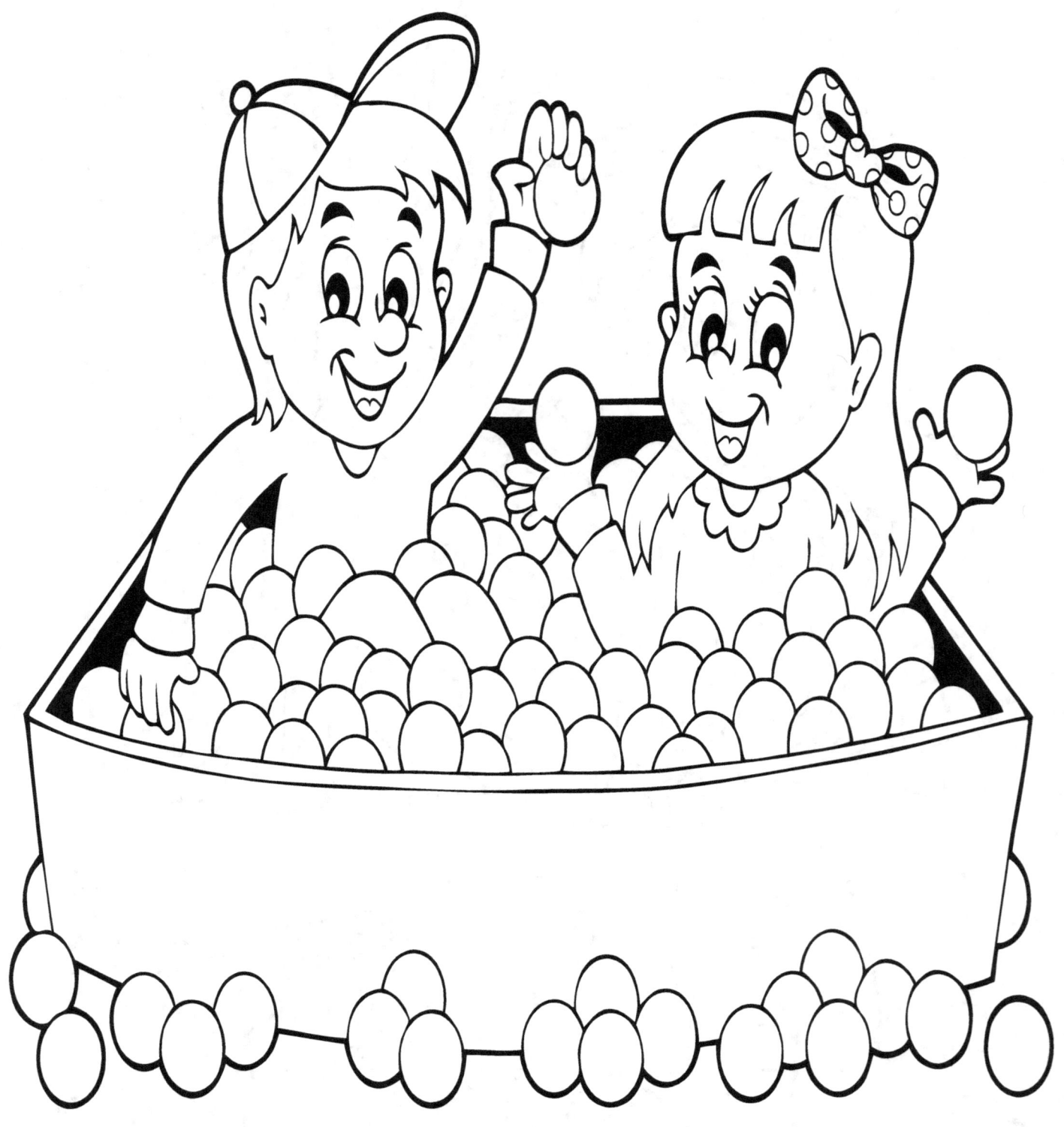

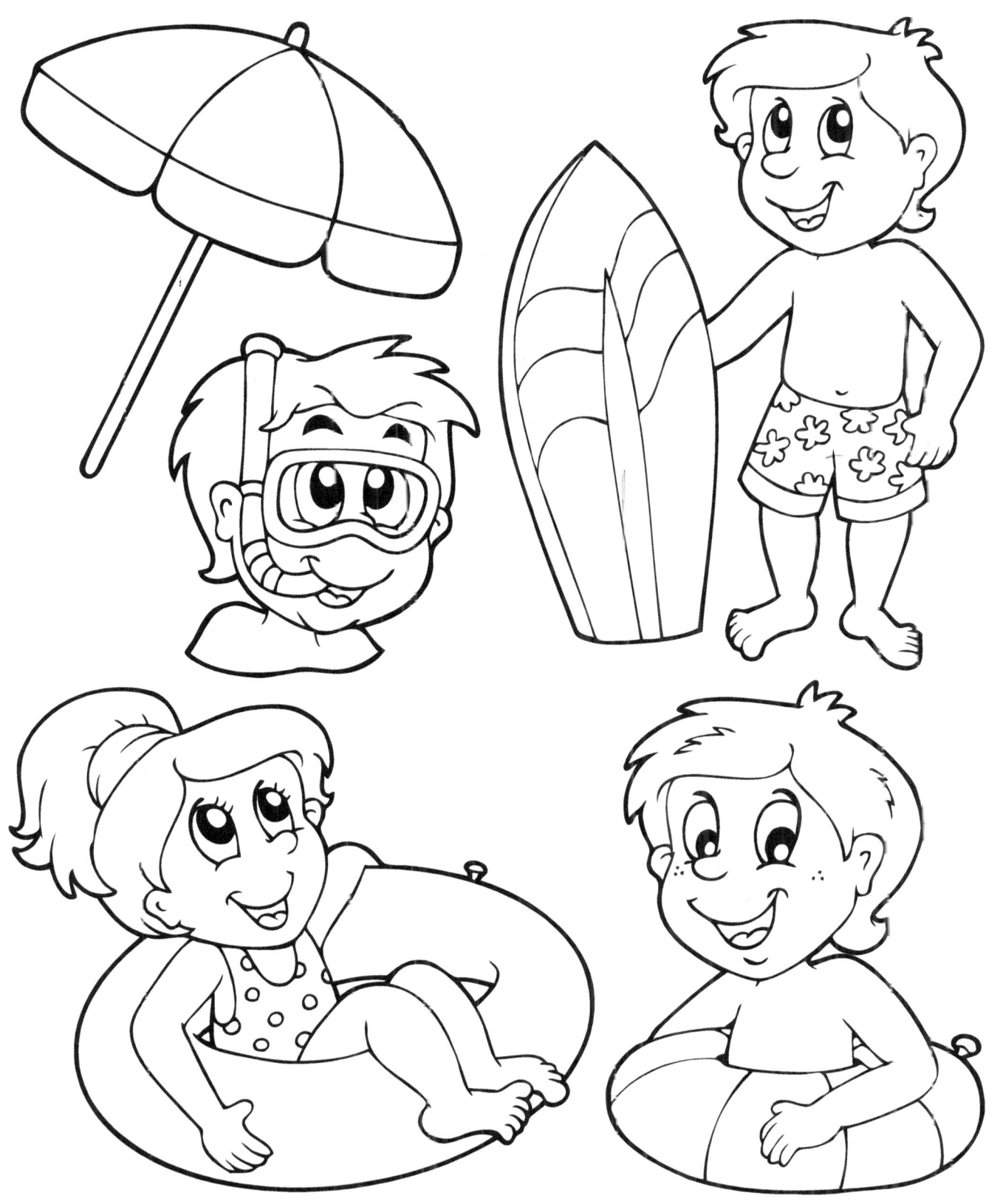

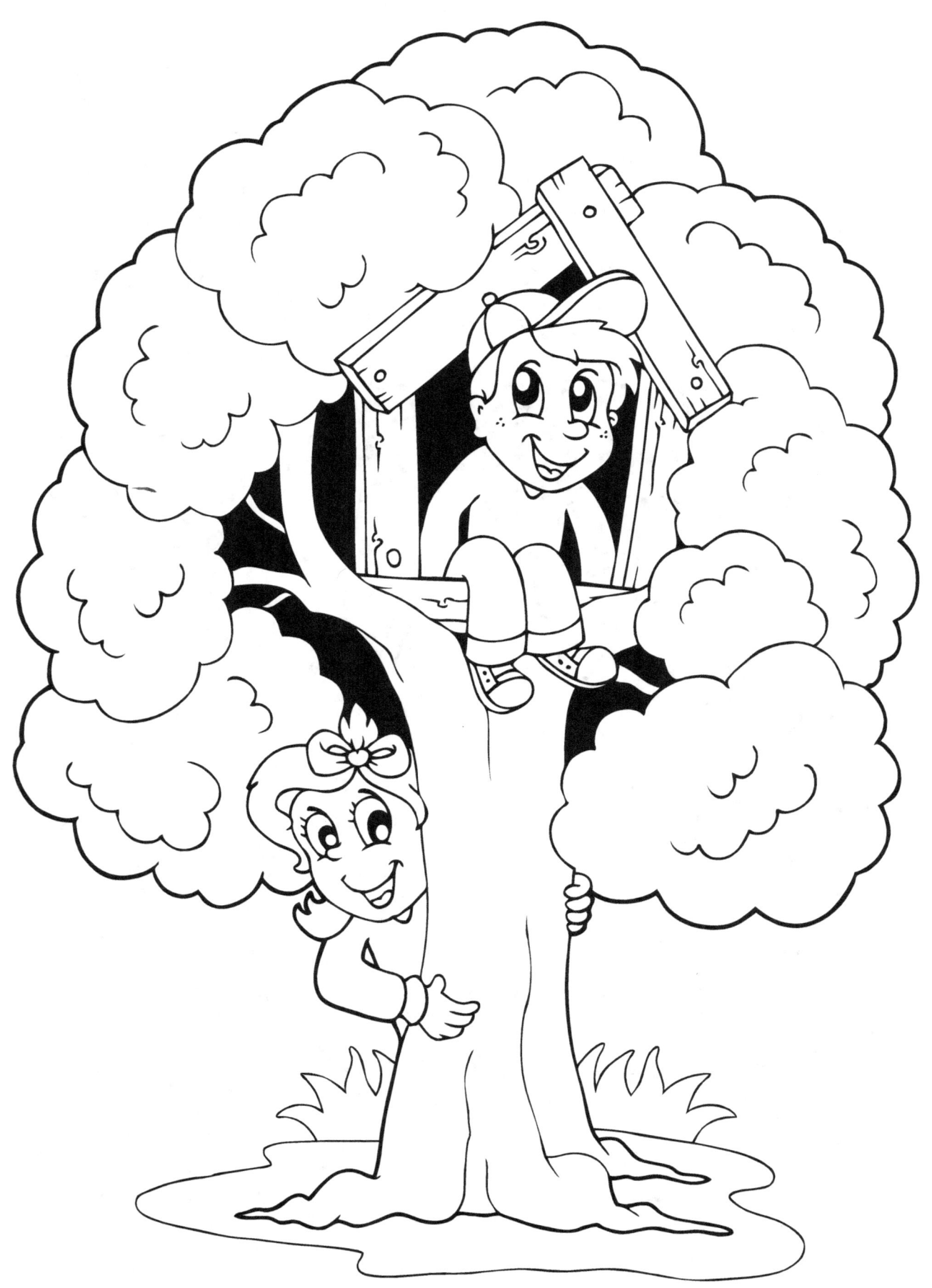

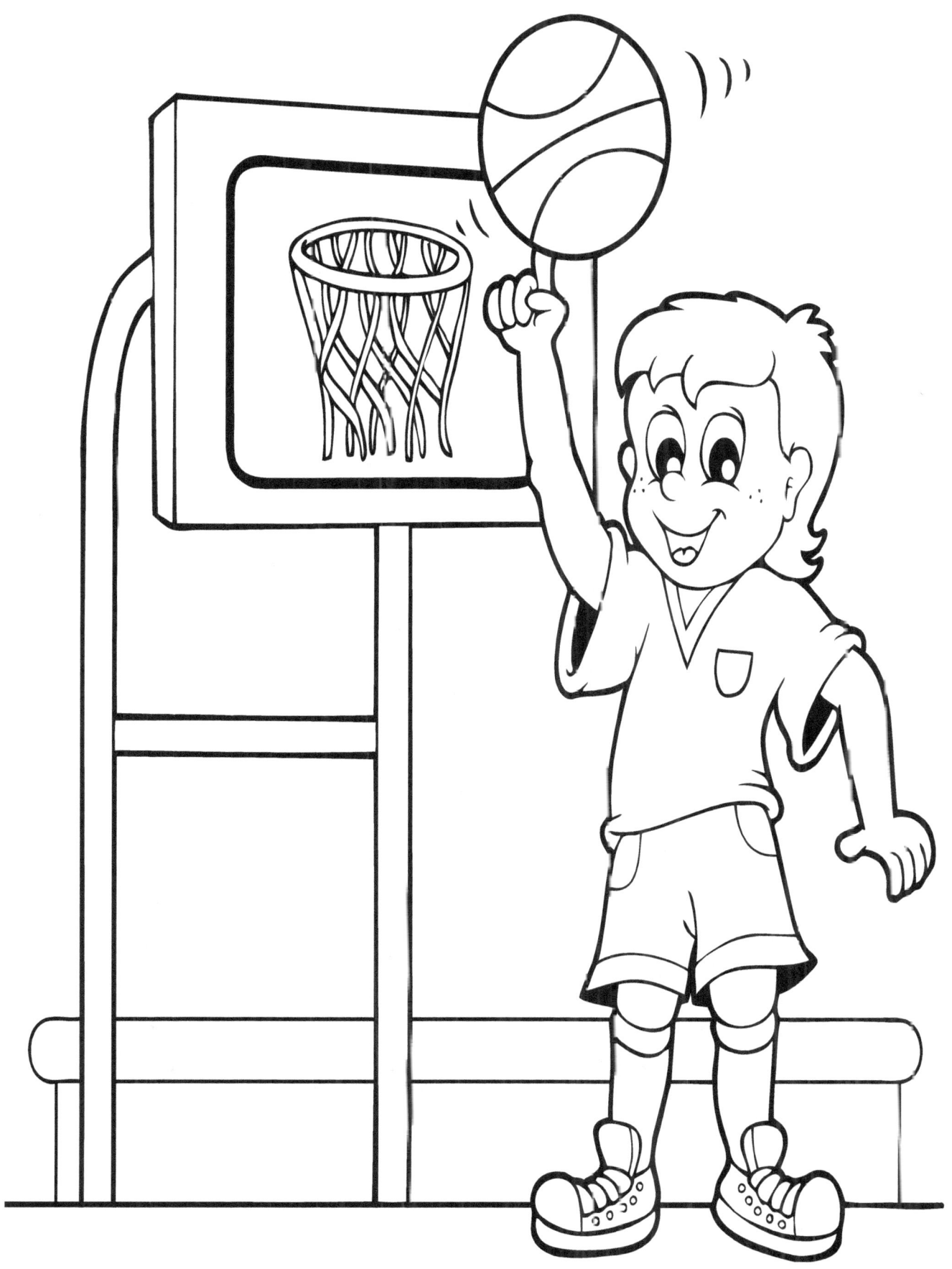

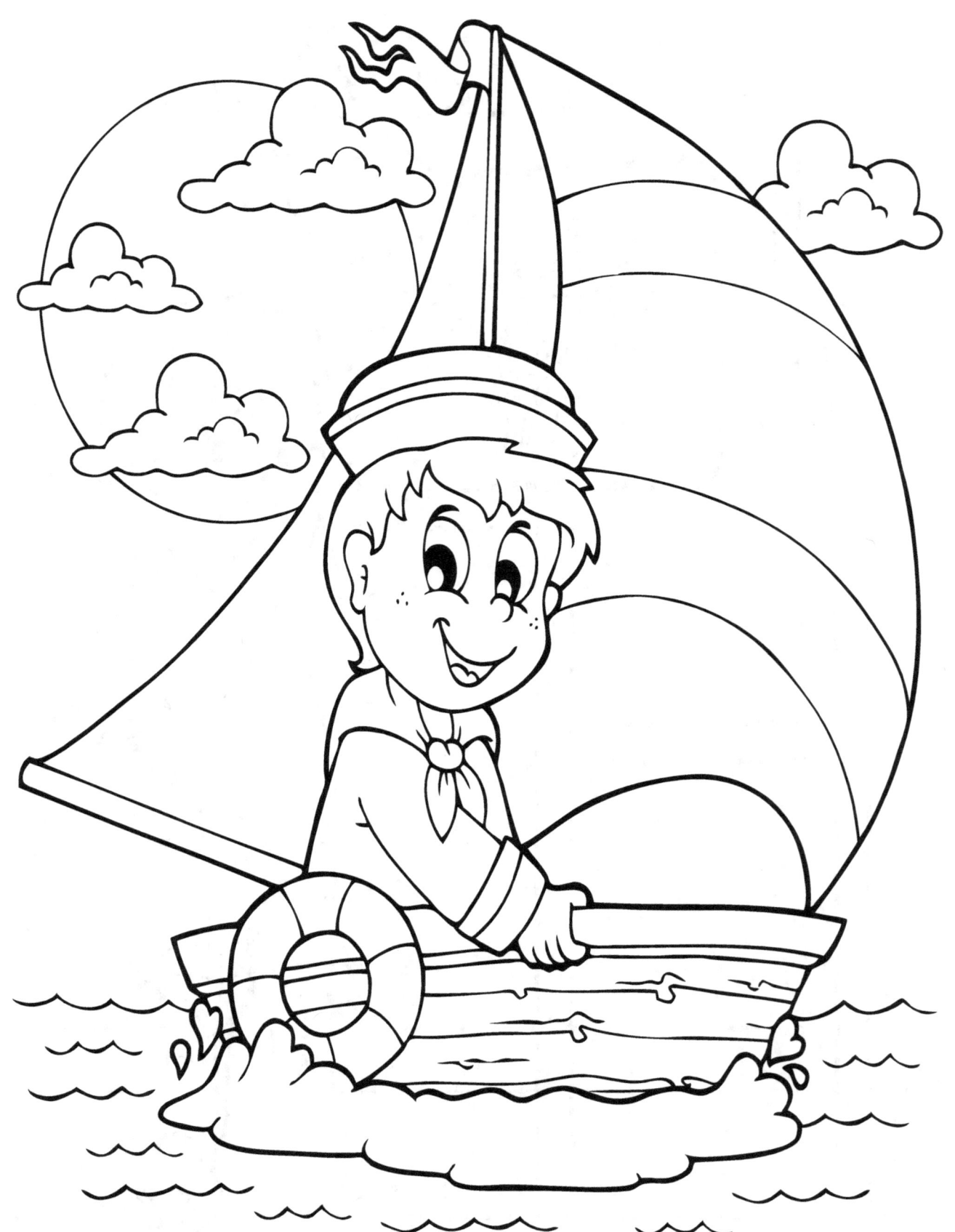

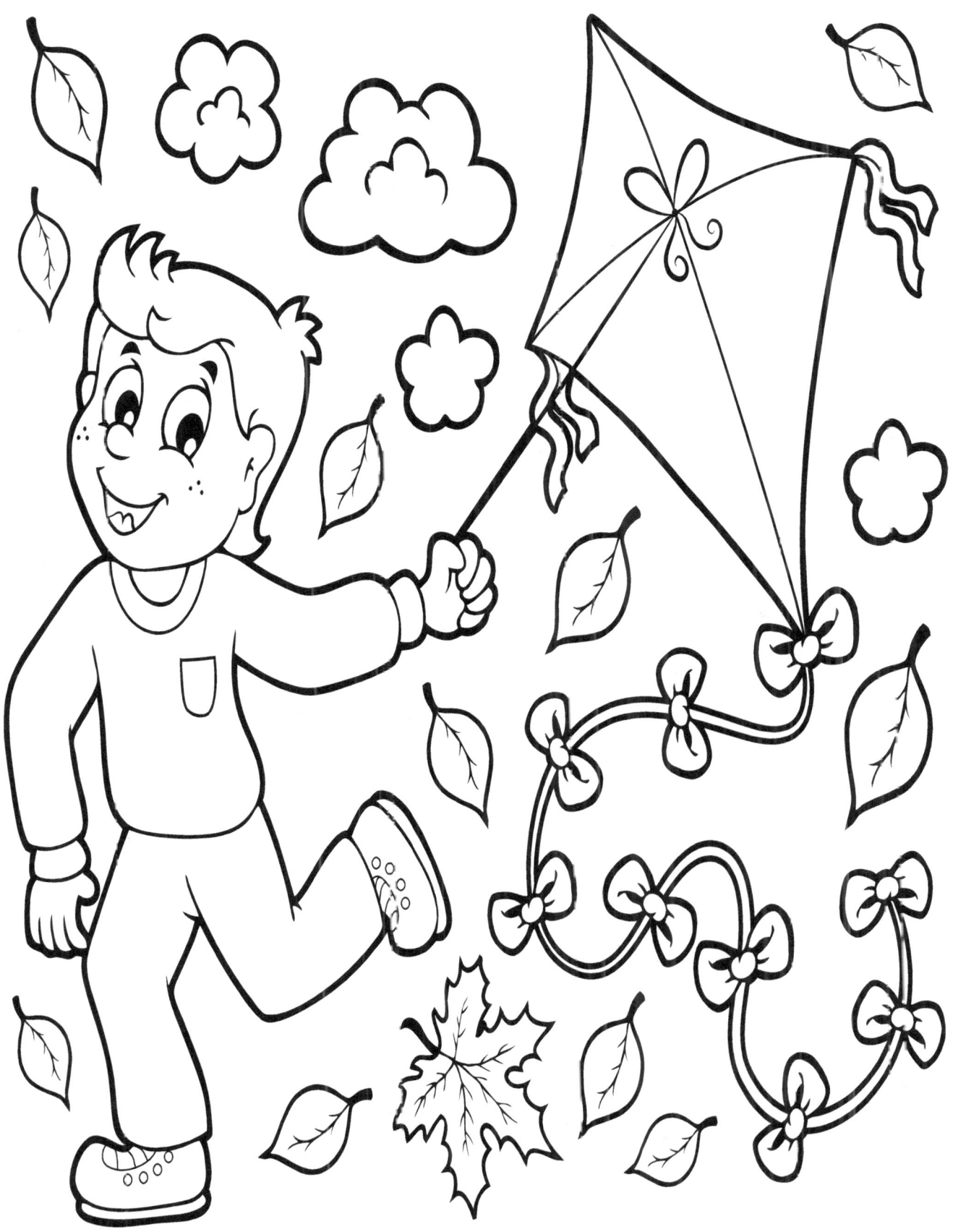

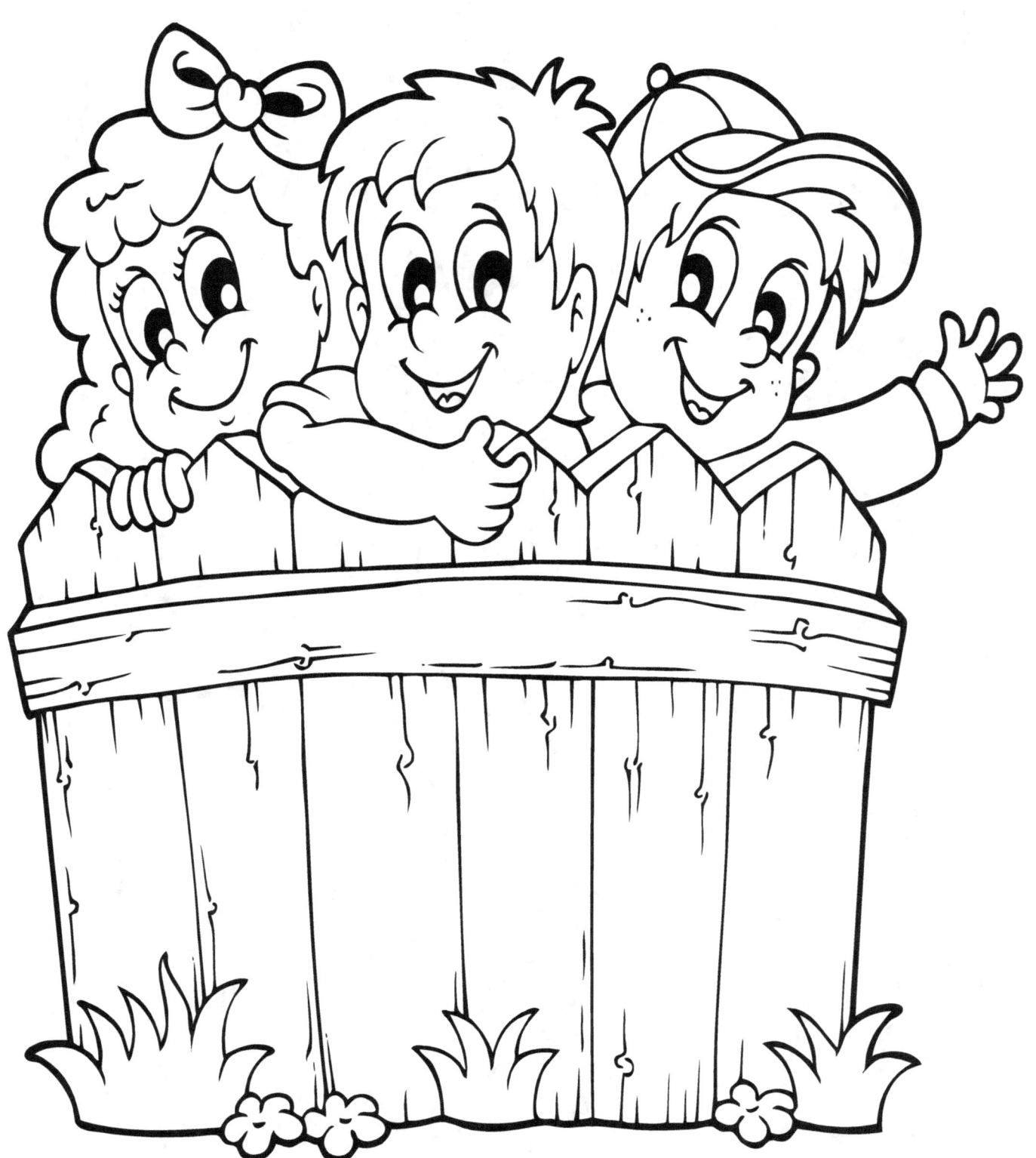

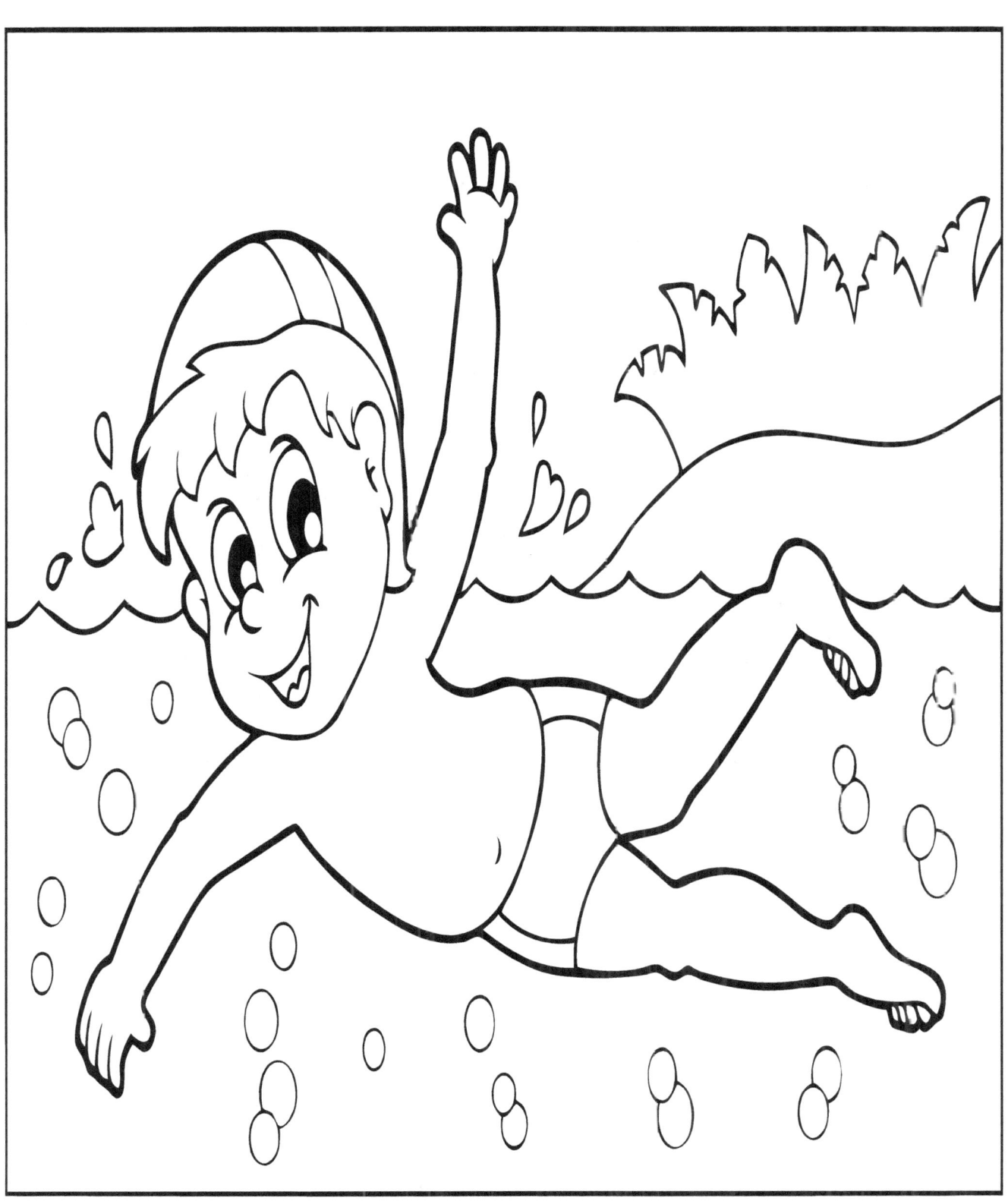

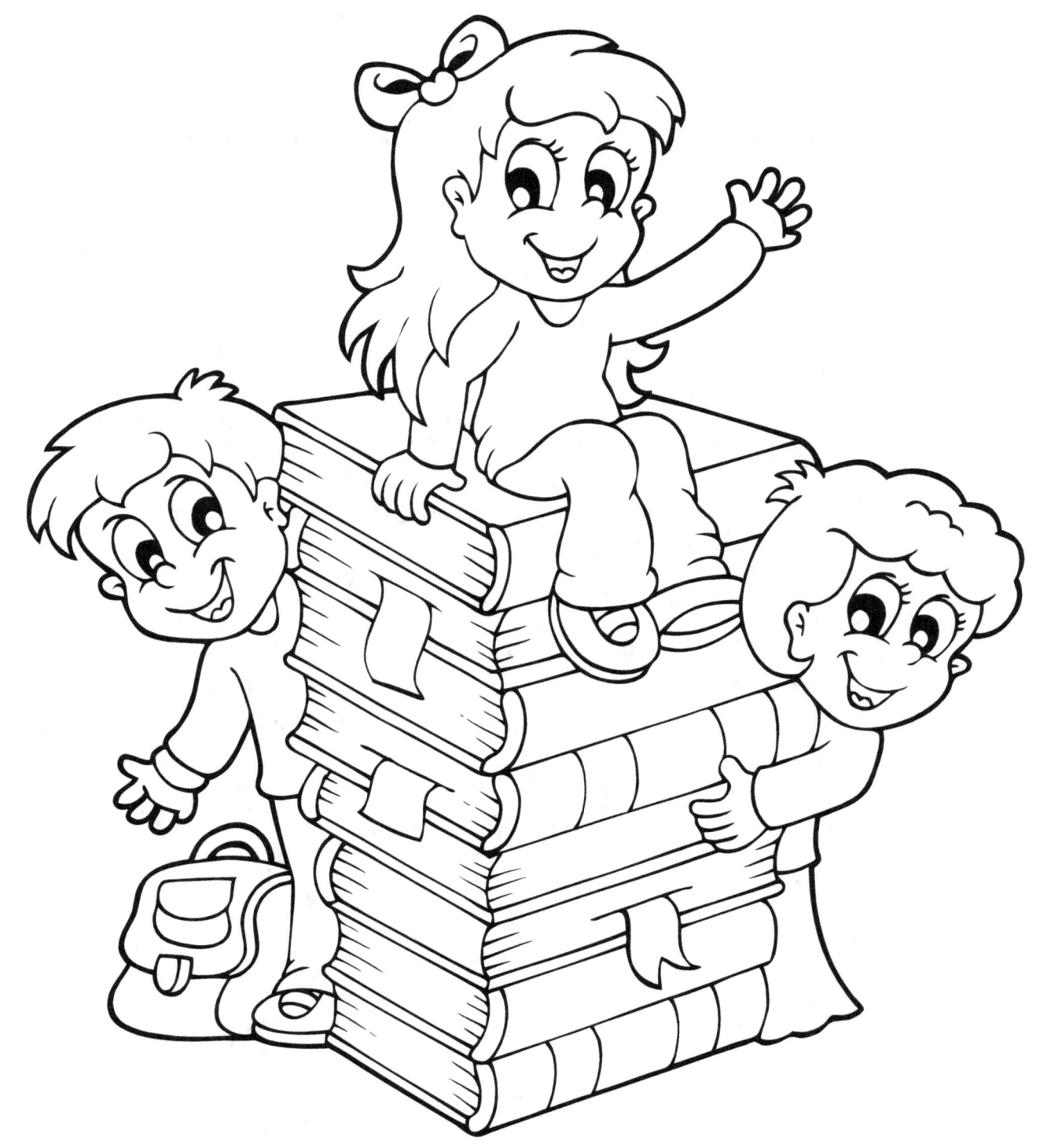

ADVENTURE LEARNING PRESS

adventurelearningpress.com
adventurelearningpress@gmail.com